PEAK PERFORMANCE:

Past, Present and Future Athletes

D1711226

You Can Always Be Better

By Nadege Beauvoir
Cheer Tumbling Dynamics Inc.

ISBN 978-0615942193

Printed in the United States of America

DEDICATION

I would like to dedicate this book to my past teammates Ken Comia and Marcus Bush and to my past and current athletes who have all inspired me to write this book on their behalf. I want nothing more then for athletes and athletic enthusiasts to have a strong starting point to leading a healthier and more fulfilling life in all that they do.

I would like to also thank my family, especially my mom and sister Marie Lege Berube and Michele Beauvoir for always believing and encouraging me to do what I love most in life, which is to spread the joys of life through excellent performance and sound nutrition.

DISCLAIMER

I am not a nutritionist. The foods I mention have been recommended to me by various health professionals for a healthy, disease-free lifestyle. These examples should be used as an overview of what can be good for you and not what you should eat specifically. I am allergic to all dairy so my dietary choices are based on 1,500 caloric intake for my blood type based upon advice from my own personal physician, Dr. Nicole Beauvoir. This book will serve as a general guideline for you to consider but you will need to find the specific diet that is right for you.

TABLE OF CONTENTS

Obstacles don't have to stop you. If you run into a wall, don't turn around and give up. Figure out how to climb it, go through it, or work around it.

— MICHAEL JORDAN

PREFACE

I have spent my life in the world of the athletes: I was a state champion in cheerleading at the high school level, and a national All Star Level 6 champion at the college level. In high school, I was heavily involved in track, gymnastics and a variety of other competitive sports, too. Currently I own a cheerleading consulting company in Illinois, which provides services such as choreography, camps, clinics and team training. I coach more than 40 private lessons per week, judge competitions, and train high school cheerleading programs.

As a former athlete turned work-obsessed, always on the go, and high-energy adult, I personally know the importance of healthy choices. I would never have been a successful athlete in my youth and definitely couldn't keep up with my demanding schedule as an adult without fully understanding how my body reacts and performs by how I fuel it.

I have built my share of great athletes over the last 14 years. No question, I am immersed in the world of athletes and healthy living. I believe that healthy choices in our lives lead to strong minds and bodies, which are motivated and powerful. I have specialized knowledge that applies to athletes who tumble and cheer, but this knowledge applies to ALL athletes, young and old alike.

I decided to share my knowledge, including easy steps, tips and real stories to put you on a good path. I want to help you become a better athlete and a better person for life! I am passionate about the subject!

I have trained some of the best, and improved some of the worst athletes. I witness each and every day how a well-maintained body and a motivated spirit creates winners, truly strong athletes at peak performance; and how a poor diet, lifestyle choices or unclear goals can lead to poor performance.

"Peak Performance" serves as a springboard that can launch you into greater health, discipline and mastery over your body and your art. Maybe you have some good habits but still feel tired, experience too many injuries, or doubt yourself. Maybe you have horrible eating habits and no discipline but get by because of natural talent. This book will help move you in the right direction, or improve you from where you are. In fact, I hope you will see this book as your personal Call-to-Action!

YOU CAN BE GREAT; YOU CAN BE BETTER, HEALTHIER AND STRONGER!

Preface

The truth of the matter is, to get to where you want to be solely depends on how much you are willing to dedicate of yourself. This is something you should know and should never forget:

You are the beginning and ending of your greatness. You can achieve whatever you want to achieve.

Let's get started!

— Nadege Beauvoir

"It doesn't matter who you are, where you come from. The ability to triumph begins with you. Always."
— OPRAH WINFREY

"Go confidently in the direction of your dreams. Live the life you have imagined."
— HENRY DAVID THOREAU

"All women are created equal...then a few become cheerleaders!"
— ERICA GARDNER, CHEER COACH

"The difference between the impossible and the possible lies in a man's determination."
— MIKE DITKA

MY STORY

There are turning points in our lives, moments when our hearts beat a mile a minute and there are too many butterflies in the stomach. I was reaching a defining moment the year my high school teammates and I competed for the State Championship in the coed varsity division of cheerleading. This was definitely a turning point for me and for my teammates: would we win after all of our hard work and reach the goal we had focused on for more than a year?

Moments before the announcement of who would win the championship, our team of ten boys and girls and two male coaches representing Maine East High School were trying everything to calm our nerves. We had trained and practiced incredibly hard for a year, we supported each other through thick and thin, and now we had performed exceptionally well. With prayers spoken, hands interlocked, heads bowed, all we could do now was wait and hope. We sat in our tight circle with our palms sweaty, tears rolling, make-up running, and hands losing feeling from holding each other's so tightly.

The last time our high school had won a championship was six years prior, when the Maine East High School coed cheer team was awarded the state prize for the first time in the history of Illinois cheerleading. A very diverse school, with over 70 countries of the world represented and an equivalent amount of languages spoken, Maine East High School was best known for its famous alumni, Harrison Ford and Hillary Rodham Clinton.

If someone had told me years before that I had a chance to become a state cheerleading champion, I would not have believed them. I had limited myself mentally and had no expectations when I was younger. I joined cheerleading in junior high school because I wanted to wear the uniform and because I also had unparalleled tumbling skills. The junior high school administration's support was lukewarm. My coach was all my teammates and I had.

As my heart fluttered at the state competition, and as each runner up was announced, thoughts that went through my head ran the gamut from the intense training we had done as a group to my algebra test earlier that week to the shooting pain coming from my injured wrist and tears flowing from my eyes. I also thought about my teammates. I truly believe I inspired them. I always pushed through my pain and tears. I worked so hard in *and* out of practice. I believed they noticed. We actually inspired each other, with teammates learning each other's story about why he or she had joined cheerleading.

We discovered the reality of just *HOW MUCH* effort went into each individuals' training and execution. The strength and dedication of each individual added up to a strong team who believed in each other. Mentally and physically, we were focused. We cared about being the best we could be, and we put everything into our performances. I think this team was one of the best I have ever worked with.

And then the announcer's warbled message came over the speaker: "The State Champions in the coed varsity division... Maine East High School!"

It took a few minutes to sink in! But it was true! As the announcer repeated those magic words and reminded us that we had a trophy to claim, I think we finally realized what had happened. With teammates and coaches converging on each other from every direction, it took a while before we got to the champions' podium. Our team and coaches, all of whom worked very hard over the past season, were rewarded that coveted championship. And we brought Maine East High School once again into the spotlight for the many accolades it deserved.

Bets had gone around the school that our program would never amount to anything. We shut down the naysayers by working hard, believing in ourselves, winning the competition. We brought back a gigantic trophy as a lasting reminder to them of our achievement. *That is when I learned I would need to rely on myself for motivation. Inspiration comes from within.* To this day I meditate often to maintain that inner peace and a sound mind.

I am Nadege Beauvoir, former Illinois State and National level all-star champion. I own a full service cheerleading company in Illinois and remain very much involved in the world of cheer and tumbling.

As I wrote in the Preface, this book is rooted in years of experience and brings information to <u>any athlete</u> looking to maximize their performance--and specifically to cheerleading athletes working to become the best cheerleaders they can be. <u>By living a healthy lifestyle and dedicating the necessary time and discipline to your sport and your life, your aims can and will be achieved.</u> My goal is to improve our communities by encouraging athletes to be healthier individuals through conscientious habits and nutritional practices. In my high school years, I was on both track and cheerleading teams. I found my track coaches put more value on nutritional practices than did my cheerleading coaches. I started to learn to eat better from them...I ate junk before that! Suggestions of what to eat before meets and practices were always discussed among track members. Conversely, those conversations were noticeably absent during my cheerleading practices.

Times have changed and now cheerleading has become so competitive that the idea of participating in multiple sports is no longer likely to be a feasible option. As it is, my desire is to apply what I learned about proper eating from my higher education degree and other disciplines from track to the sport of cheerleading. I now work with athletes of various levels and skill sets throughout Illinois school and park district programs. What I know to be true is that the experiences we get during our adolescent years are critical to our overall development as adults.

I have covered three main areas in this book on Peak Performance, which apply to all athletes:

Food and Fuel for your Body (Chapters 1 – 4)

Practice Makes Perfect! (Chapter 5)

Attitude and Inner Strength (Chapter 6)

Try my advice. You will definitely notice a positive change and become a better performer and competitor. And the changes will stay with you for the rest of your life.

"Knowing is not enough, we must apply. Willing is not enough, we must do."

— BRUCE LEE

CHAPTER 1

FOOD & PERSONAL CHOICES "TAKING CONTROL!"

How can I become a better athlete? What do I need to know, and what can I change today? What are the secrets?

These are typical questions that students ask me all the time.

Let's start with the basics: you can make or break your game with the food you eat. Also remember the old saying, "You are what you eat."

You have one body, and that body depends on your choices and how you care for it. It depends on the fuel of sound food and liquids to help you think better, compete better and stay healthy.

- Good food and drink makes your body strong.

- Good food makes your skin look good!

- The right amount of food in combination with your exercise and training keeps your body at its best weight and peak performance.

- You look good in your clothes and competition uniforms.

- With good food and drink, your energy lasts longer and you don't crash.

WHAT'S THE ALTERNATIVE?

Eat and drink bad foods, and:

- You won't have sustainable energy.

- You will get sick easier.

- You won't be as strong, including muscle strength.

- You won't feel as good.

- You won't look as good (skin, hair, body).

- You won't operate at peak performance.

- You will not be the competitor you should be.

Scarf down those burgers and fries after a practice because you didn't eat properly before, and you have not only eaten too many calories but have eaten foods that will NOT optimize your muscles and body.

Keep drinking those sodas all day, and minerals and nutrients will be sucked from your body and your bones will become less strong. Plus you will be more likely to have sugar crashes and run out of energy.

Keep skipping breakfast and feel horrible.

Keep being lazy about your body, and you will never reach your real potential.

You will not be in optimal form, and you will not be competitive. Other girls, those that are eating well and at the right time, practicing, and taking control of their life will beat you.

> *"Take care of your body;*
> *it's the only place you have to live!"*
> — JIM ROHN

Did you ever compare two older people of the same age: one who eats good foods but doesn't overeat, one who has exercised during her life and made good choices (like not smoking) compared to the one who eats fast food and junk, drinks colas all day, never cared about exercise or good living? There is a clear and visual difference! You don't notice these affects so much when you are young, but bad choices will catch up with you and good choices will sustain you!

Here is something you WILL notice right now. Teams that eat right and eat at the right time will be stronger and be better competitors against teams that do not. Are you the team that is dedicated and eats right, or not? If not, follow my simple guidelines, get on the right track and you will see the improvements!

It is as simple as this:

What you eat determines how much energy you will have to burn during practices and competitions, and how long that energy will last.

I work with athletes intensively on a daily and even hourly basis, and have worked with many through the years. This has given me good insight (along with my own experience) to assess what an athlete needs and factors that contribute directly to performance improvement. I've worked out weekly eating schedules with students and their parents to ensure they can peak their performance through great nutritional choices – and overcome their previous poor choices.

I can tell you there is nothing more powerful than a motivated athlete. I have witnessed the changes in the kids who cleaned up their acts and the new energy and motivation they have! I give them credit for their hard work, because they were the ones who made the choice to become better. An important reward is improvement of current skills and the ability to move forward to new ones.

So when students ask me, *"Does it really matter what I eat?"*... the answer is *"Yes, it definitely matters!"*

REPLENISHING YOUR MUSCLES

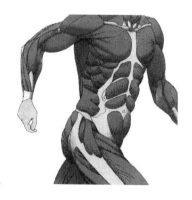

It takes time to replenish your muscles. There are several ways to do this. One is to eat right *the night before* a practice or competition, with whole grains and other nutritionally sound foods to properly fuel your muscles. This is done in much the same way as one fuels a vehicle with gas in order to drive it. You must be aware of what you are putting into your body if you expect favorable results.

Quite often, athletes' performance is *limited* by poor nutritional habits due to a lack of education, dietary extremism and a lack of meal preparation practicality (or even laziness.) Your busy lifestyle can also lean you towards fast food that won't complement your true needs. Finding a way to blend practicality with convenience becomes a must for your food and drink choices.

This leads me to the first rule.

RULE #1: It is absolutely necessary to take control of what I put into my body.

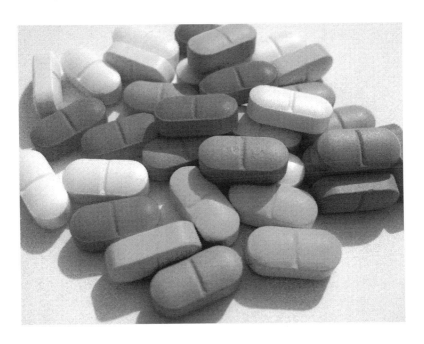

Outside commercial media will NOT assist you in this. In fact, a study published in <u>Nutrition, Dietary Supplements, and Nutriceuticals</u>[1] found that 80-90% of commercial television advertising directed toward youth is for processed, unhealthy foods found in grocery stores and fast food restaurants. The success of these ads' influence is closely associated with the risk and rise in childhood obesity.

Even schools may not properly direct youth toward healthy nutritional choices. In a study of 395 American public schools, 82% of middle schools and 97% of high schools carried vending machines for student use. Five out of six of these machines sold low nutrient foods to those students, sending a subtle message to them that these foods are beneficial to their well-being being that they are offered in educational spaces.

Two of my very talented students, Katie and Lindsey, are extraordinary athletes. They started tumbling with me in elementary school, and soon after puberty they both started becoming less focused and less energetic. I sat down with them to talk about what they ate and talked to their moms. Their diets were not good. I put together a food plan that would be healthier and improve their energy and performance.

<u>The very next week, both Katie and Lindsey reported that they had 50% more energy and stamina</u> during their lessons and in practices. Because they felt more alert and stronger, they performed better in the gym *and* in the classroom. They were sold on the new, healthier approach and while they were both already talented athletes, there was marked improvement. Katie and Lindsey both worked on the weekly grocery list for their families and took control of what they ate, which also benefitted their families.

Lindsey (who is 15 years old at the time I am writing this), says:

"I do believe nutrition makes a difference because when I eat something healthy like an apple, I feel more energized and when I eat something higher in fat, I feel more drowsy and low energy. It affects my performance...Now, good nutrition has become a life decision for me."

RULE #2: I must be willing to make a change and some new choices. I must be willing to break out of my old habits.

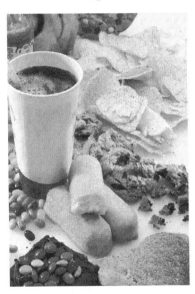 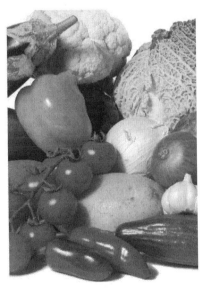

You are the one who decides what you will eat, and you can make choices of better foods over poor foods. You will learn and then decide *when* the best time is to eat certain foods for optimal performance – so you won't want to run to

McDonald's after a practice because you are starving, or eat a candy bar and then have a sugar crash.

You don't have to get rid of all foods that you love. There are healthy alternatives for practically all of your guilty pleasures, which I cover throughout the book. As mentioned before, however, eating right is a lifestyle choice.

Are you a dedicated athlete? If you are, you must be willing to make a change to be competitive in athletics and serious about a strong body.

SOME REAL EXAMPLES

Some of my students were asked to name five or six foods they choose to eat regularly, which have replaced bad foods in their lives:

Jade, whose cheer squad placed at State at the Icca State Championship competition (and who was a conference champion in volleyball and track), says:

> Apples, strawberries, clif bars, fish and pasta.

Kaitlyn, whose cheer squad won first at every competition it entered and placed top 10 at State, says:

> Apples, carrots, steak, pasta and healthy cereal. No sugary drinks.

Leanna, who has placed top 3 in cheer competition, says:

> Carrots, green beans, bananas, yogurt, chicken and wheat bread.

<u>Brianna</u>, who has placed at State Championships, says:

> Zucchini, broccoli, almonds, Romaine lettuce and pomegranates.

<u>Sara-Anne</u>, who has won several athletic championship titles in synchronized skating, cheerleading and swimming, says:

> Green vegetables, blueberries, oatmeal, chicken, white fish and milk.

<u>Katie</u> who has won several regional and national cheerleading championship titles both at the all star and high school level, is also a champion skater and swimmer says:

> Apples, bananas, broccoli and ALL fruits and vegetables!

Why don't you write down four bad foods that you eat, and what you could replace them with. There are more suggestions and ideas in the next chapters on good foods, if you need help:

BAD FOODS I EAT   **GOOD FOODS I WILL START TO EAT**

1. _____   1. _____

2. _____   2. _____

3. _____   3. _____

4. _____   4. _____

About her Diet, Leanna says,

> "In the morning, I eat a breakfast bar or protein drink because it allows me to feel good. For lunch, I have a sandwich with yogurt (I only eat chicken) and some fruit. I'll have a snack of cheese and fruit in the afternoon. Dinner is always something different."

About her Food Choices, Brianna says:

> "I eat toast with peanut butter or cereal with berries for breakfast. I'll have a salad with chicken, lettuce, spinach, cucumbers, carrots with baked pita chips, fruit and a small sweet for lunch. For dinners, I eat a meat, a starch and a vegetable. I drink 51 - 68 ounces of water a day."

Before we move on to discuss timing of foods in the next chapter, let's look at a summary of the Rules so far:

▸ *RULE #1: It is absolutely necessary to take control of what I put into my body.*

▸ *RULE #2: I must be willing to make a change and some new choices. I must be willing to break out of my old habits.*

"If you don't do what's ideal for your body, you're the one who comes up on the short end."

— JULIUS ERVING

CHAPTER 2

FOOD AND DRINK "TIMING IS EVERYTHING!"

In this chapter, I will let you in on something that is very important but that isn't commonly talked about: timing of your meals and how to properly fuel your muscles.

LET'S TALK ABOUT WHEN I SHOULD EAT

Before I go into details about *what* kinds of food and drink your body needs (covered in Chapter 4), I want to talk about *when* you should eat first.

You will soon see how timing is everything to competing athletes and then the food types will make more sense.

Time, patience and determination can accomplish wonders. Remember, the food you eat can make or break your game.

RULE #3: Ideally, I will eat five times a day roughly totaling a 2,200 to 2,500 caloric intake. I can make or break my game with the food I eat!

If you are not already eating like this, I would recommend that instead of increasing how much you are eating now, take the same amount and spread it into five meals. Why? You are using up much energy during the day but often only eat a few meals. That approach does not sustain energy or nourish your body properly. <u>By spreading meals through the day, your body is nourished more properly</u>. This does not mean five full meals, but typically three meals and two healthy snacks.

RULE #4: Eat well the night before and 3 hours before a practice or a competition to eliminate fatigue, lack of physical strength and undernourished muscles.

Preparation for game-time should begin three to four hours before any event to allow for the very best digestion process and ongoing energy supply. According to J. Anderson, L. Young and S. Prior writing for Colorado State University Extension program, those pre-game meals <u>should be high in starch</u> due to your body's ability to break starches down easier than proteins or fats. Cold cereals, pastas and/or breads otherwise known as complex carbohydrates are among this group. Fruits and vegetables are also a go-to in these cases.

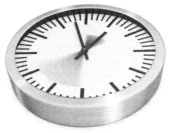

All of these foods will digest at an even rate to provide you with consistent energy and will empty from the stomach in two to three hours. <u>With little time left on the clock, two to three hours before an event, many athletes will opt for a liquid diet.</u> This will move out of the stomach by game time and, depending on the nature of the meal, have your body properly nourished and ready to go. This can and should be a carb-based drink that also contains some protein.

A familiar choice is chocolate milk or vegetable smoothies. A number of common, retail-ready smoothies fill these needs but, time allowing, you can easily make your own with your favorite fruits, nuts and vegetables in a blender.

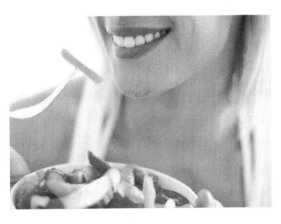

Eating three to four hours before practice will supply your mind and muscles with the right amount of energy sources and give your body time for untroubled digestion.

Student Sara-Anne says, "I used to never eat before practices, especially in the morning, but I found myself not quite awake and I was worn out by the first hour. I learned to eat an hour before practice, and then I had much more energy."

<u>I will talk more about carbohydrates and proteins, but know this -- they are your muscles' friends.</u> Eat brown pastas and/or grains and other foods recommended by your doctor or dietician. Try salmon, tilapia, and other fish choices or

multigrain noodle lasagna stuffed with lean meat fillings. Incorporate plenty of vegetables and herbs for energy and overall nutrition. Also include vegetable smoothies and drink plenty of water the night before a practice or event.

Here is what Brianna says, *"If I don't eat before practice, I feel sluggish and can't stop yawning. I usually can't stop thinking about what I am GOING to eat, which distracts me from the task at hand. I almost always eat before practice, but not too much!"*

AFTER PRACTICE OR A COMPETITION

You will find that what you consume *after* practice or competition is just as important as what you consume beforehand, which leads us to the next rule.

RULE #5: After the hard work of a competition or workout, I will eat a small meal within thirty minutes of completion to replenish my muscles and energy stores (for better recovery.)

This is very necessary.

Make this meal a mix of carbohydrates, proteins and fats. The carbs will replenish diminished glycogen stores (translated simply as *muscle food*) and the proteins will synthesize best within the body at this time. You want to refuel your exerted muscles so they may smoothly recover from the day's work, therefore allowing you to better prepare for

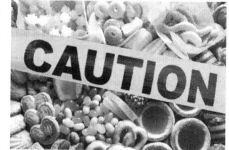

your next practice or competition. This will be discussed in further detail.

Listen, many young athletes work hard at competition or practice, don't nourish themselves at the right time and then they are starving. But why would you burn 700 calories only to take in 2500 in one meal? Quit it with all the fast food burgers, fries and colas if you are serious about being a better you.

RULE #6: Plan Ahead!

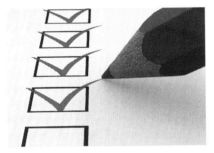
Here is what happened to me, when I discovered the changes I needed in my diet. I would start out buying all of these healthy foods, and then I would get busy and forget about them, or go back to my old ways of junk food because I didn't plan ahead. I had good intentions but didn't follow through. Then I got creative and created a routine. I planned ahead!

I would buy the healthy groceries on a day that I had less to do and then I would chop up the fruits and veggies and use my blender to create 5 cups of a smoothie. I would put these cups in the freezer. Then at night before I went to bed, I would put one in the fridge so that in the morning, it was ready and I could drink it on the way to school.

When I realized I was feeling better every morning, I started to plan all of my meals ahead! I planned ahead and made my lettuce wrap and package my snacks the night before, and took them to school. I was able to avoid junk food because I planned.

Even now, years later, I stick to this discipline and my weight does not fluctuate and I remain a very high energy person. Sometimes I work in the gym 12 hours a day, but I constantly fuel my body with the nutritious foods that I have planned for.

I help the students I coach to plan ahead. For instance, I have them bring three cliff bars with them during a competitive event: one for arrival, one for an hour prior to competition, and one for immediately after competition.

HINT

Look to your favorite celebrity or athlete for inspiration – most of them eat a very healthy and balanced diet to maintain their looks and energy. Find motivation wherever you can and from anyone, but find it! Don't waste another day!

ADVICE

Plan your meals, plan ahead for your breaks and time after practice. Keep a protein bar, carrot sticks, fruit, low salt pretzels, or half of a peanut butter sandwich in your bag to eat on a break during or after practice. Find what you like, make lists and get to know what is best for you – and then just do it! As I mention later, your team could designate an empty locker for healthy snacks. Just don't be starving and then eat the worst possible foods or drinks. Care for your body and it will care for you.

<u>Here is what Sara-Ann says</u>, *"Once I started to concentrate on the foods I ate, I felt that I had so much more energy and felt lighter on my toes, which is really important for tumbling and cheerleading. I also didn't feel as worn out after practices or private training sessions."*

Make it fun, become a better athlete and feel better!

We are going to take a look at actual food suggestions and more information in the next chapter, but let's review the rules in this chapter:

▶ *RULE #3: Ideally, I will eat five times a day roughly totaling a 2,200 to 2,500 caloric intake. I can make or break my game with the food I eat!*

▶ *RULE #4: Eat well the night before and 3 hours before a practice or a competition to eliminate fatigue, lack of physical strength and undernourished muscles.*

▶ *RULE #5: After the hard work of a competition or workout, I will eat a small meal within thirty minutes of completion to replenish my muscles and energy stores (for better recovery.)*

▶ *RULE #6: Plan Ahead!*

"Making a true decision means committing to achieving a result, and then cutting yourself off from any other possibility."

— TONY ROBBINS

CHAPTER 3

WHAT TO EAT
"YOU ARE WHAT YOU EAT!"

I will say this again, because it is important: "You are what you eat!"

If you want to be a top-performing athlete, and if you want to be the best you can be, you must eat nourishing foods. Do you want to be mediocre? Do you want to hold yourself back? Then keep eating junk. It is a choice, and you can make this choice!

LET'S TALK ABOUT <u>WHAT</u> SHOULD I EAT AND DRINK

<u>More than half of what you eat daily should be fruits and vegetables</u>. Eating these live, uncooked (and sometimes cooked) natural foods enhances your body and brings the natural nutrients to your body.

It has been proven that eating raw blended vegetables provides you with *more natural energy* than coffee and lifts

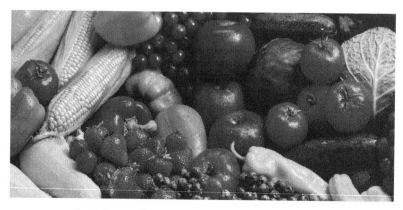

your mood without the energy "crash" commonly associated with caffeine or sugar. A healthy intake of fruits and vegetables is essential for good health.

WHAT IF I AM NOT EATING FRUITS AND VEGETABLES?

If you aren't eating many now, <u>start working them into your diet</u>. Again, make it fun. Go to the grocery store or farmer's market, look at the great choices, start with ones that seem appealing to you. Sample and taste. Once you start to eat more fruits and vegetables, you will start to feel better and more energetic. Your skin will look clearer and your energy will be sustainable. You'll feel good and then you'll want more!

Add more fruits and vegetables to your diet each week, and you'll soon discover the great tastes and good results. Tasty bananas or apples, for instance, are a great and easy treat; have some of those leafy greens or salad green with yummy tomatoes, cucumbers and peppers. <u>Make smoothies</u>. Cut up crunchy snacks like cucumbers and carrots. Eat seasonal fruits. Get creative! Eating some vegetables with your chicken or meat at night tastes good and is good for you. And before you know it, you will crave these foods!

You might not think about it so much today, but you will one day. Increasing the amount of fruits and vegetables you eat can help reduce the risk of many debilitating disorders, for instance, cancer, cardiovascular disease, and obesity. According to the US Department of Agriculture 60% of American adults DO NOT eat the daily, recommended level of five or more servings of fruits and vegetables. The youth statistic that met recommendations was even lower; a mere 1% of boys and 2% of girls aged 9-18 years old.

**As athletes, we must be better than those statistics.
And you can be!**

I HAVE BEEN IN YOUR SHOES

I know what I am talking about – I used to eat junk food all the time when I was young, and then into junior high. And though I was a strong, fearless athlete, I wasn't that healthy and often felt sick. Through my high school track coach, I discovered the importance of good foods and started to look into this subject more. Once I started to change my diet, and started to feel better and better, I was sold. I kept learning about nutrition and became my own expert!

MY TYPICAL DIET

In order to help you understand the kind of foods I am talking about, let me share my own diet. I also include <u>why</u> I think these choices are good and the important qualities they hold.

BREAKFAST

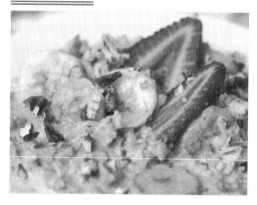

WHAT: To start my day out I'll have a bowl of oatmeal, a mug of green tea and a smoothie (one banana, 2-4 cups of frozen spinach or fresh kale, hemp or chia protein powder or flaxseed meal, frozen raspberries and blueberries, with carrot or orange juice or flax milk).

WHY: I eat **oatmeal** because it is a fat burner, curbs hunger, is high in fiber and protein, low in fat, and protects against heart disease and cancer. It stabilizes blood sugars and reduces the risk of diabetes, too.

I drink **green tea** because it lowers cholesterol, increases metabolism, and it is an antioxidant. It also reduces plaque! **Ginger tea** actually promotes proper digestion and normal blood circulation, and can help reduce menstrual cramps while boosting immunity.

The ingredients in my **smoothie** all have great qualities, too. **Spinach** and kale improves red blood cell function, is high in calcium and vitamin K and optimizes muscle use. **Carrot juice** can improve vision, skin, hair and nails (beta-carotene/Vitamin A) and reduces bile and fat in the liver. **Raspberries** are 10 times more effective at reliving inflammation than aspirin. They also may neutralize other cell-damaging substances. **Blueberries** are a powerful phytonutrient, a natural form of aspirin that reduces inflammation and combats brain diseases. **Flaxseed meal** is rich in healthy omega-3 fats, fiber and antioxidants and helps assist in absorbing sugars, while **hemp protein powder** is a complete protein more digestible than soy. It builds the immune system and lubricates arteries.

If I am craving meat I opt for one boiled or scrambled egg with one slice of turkey bacon and a smoothie. **Eggs** are low calorie high protein foods good for muscle growth and repair, and also a brain food.

I'll then take my vitamins (Multi vitamin, omega force and vitamin D supplements) and wait 2-3 hours before my next meal.

I make sure to have two full cups of room temperature or warm water before I eat again if I'm not going to participate in any physical activity in the next three hours.

LUNCH

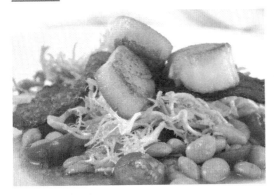

WHAT: My lunch might be a light salad or rice and fish with juice or water. Consider a lettuce wrap or sandwich for lunch, or just a vegetable smoothie containing kale or spinach, orange, raspberries, blueberries, bananas, celery, carrots, beets, ginger and water or pomegranate juice as a base.

WHY: Mixed greens will feed the bones with vitamin K and calcium. A lettuce wrap with turkey, avocado and greens will be easily digestible and give you complete proteins with all 18 amino acids. It is also anti-inflammatory. A turkey sandwich on wheat will give you a lean high protein meat, and the wheat or whole grain bread provides you fiber. Avoid white breads.

MIDDAY SNACK

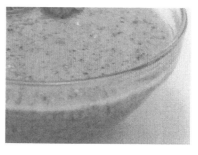

WHAT: Unsalted baked pita chips and pesto dip (with crushed garlic and crushed basil leaves sprinkled with pepper and salt to taste) or something comparable, like a granola bar with fruit, sunflower seeds, cashews, unsalted pretzels, or half of a peanut butter & jelly sandwich.

WHY: A peanut butter and jelly sandwich curbs appetite and is high in muscle-building proteins. Healthy snacks curb your appetite, nourish muscles and sustain your energy.

DINNER

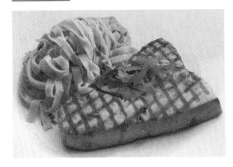

WHAT and WHY: I will eat brown rice pasta or lean steak/fish and mixed vegetables. Rice is my weakness, but I'll elect to have brown rice instead of white or substitute white mashed potatoes for vegan sweet mashed potatoes. These make for healthier options. By the way, corn pasta is excellent for those who love pasta but want to avoid allergic gluten. Salmon is a great choice for fish – it is full of heart healthy Omega 3 acids (falling 3rd behind walnuts and flaxseeds), and supports your joint cartilage. It is high in calcium, too. Your body needs proteins found in steak, and your muscles needs carbs.

DAILY VITAMINS

WHAT: Multi or prenatal Gummy Bears Vitamins, Flaxseed Oil supplements, Omega 3 6 9 Supplements, 500 milligrams of Vitamin C and Calcium with Vitamin D and Magnesium (since I don't consume dairy products).

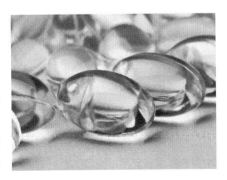

WHY: The Flaxseed and Omega vitamins enhance healthy hair, skin, and nail growth. There is no need to take more than the recommended daily amount and doing so can be dangerous.

MORE FOOD SUGGESTIONS

- Indispensable and convenient options to consider in your daily diet are peanut butter (made with non-hydrogenated oil), nuts, one egg daily, electrolyte-enhanced water and all-natural protein bars. These are just great foods to consider eating as an athlete who is constantly using their muscles and burning energy.

- Limit dairy use and choose tea instead of coffee.

- I personally like organic foods, so I do most of my food shopping at Trader Joe's because they offer affordable organic groceries. They are well known for healthier version of many snacks, reduced sugar juices, and other tasty meals. Whole Foods or other organic food stores may exist in your town.

- You need protein to stay healthy and support your muscles. When consuming meat choose lean or low-fat options when you can. Fish, nuts, and seeds contain healthy oils, so pick these foods frequently over other meats or poultry. Equipping your body with any or a combination of these protein sources before or after a workout will support muscle development and muscle repair.

- Carbohydrates, as mentioned in the section about *when* you should eat, are important to athletes... pasta is a favored carbohydrate.

- Stop drinking soda. Contrary to popular belief there is **nothing** healthy about diet sodas, colas in particular. *Consumption of soda leeches away important vitamins and minerals from your bones leaving them weakened and with unhealthy growth.*

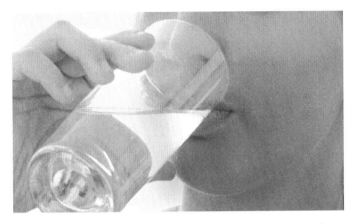

- Do drink water, and lots of it! Water is an absolute must. It has the ability to move in and outside our cells transporting vital nutrients and other substances throughout the body that complete crucial metabolic and chemical reactions and handles cell maintenance. Water regulates your body's temperature and maintains our body's structure and protection. It guards against those muscle cramps.

- Our bodies are composed of approximately 60-70% water, varying by gender and body size. It is suggested that we drink half of our weight in ounces per day to maintain that balance. (Your weight = 100lbs. You should be drinking at least 50oz of water).

- Avoid caffeine (cola, coffee) in general and definitely pre-competition as it may lead to dehydration by increasing runs to the bathroom. 100% juices, smoothies and water will assimilate faster and give your body the hydration it will need and more healthy energy to run on.

- Avoid protein or amino-acid supplementation powders and pills in place of real meals. Outside of being unnecessary, they are known to place stress on the kidneys and liver, have been linked to dehydration, unwanted weight gain and hypercalciuria (excessive calcium excretion through urination). These conditions are bad for everyone, however they are particularly detrimental for athletes. Any athlete considering consuming supplements in place of meals should consult with their doctor or dietary professional first.

WHAT DO SOME OF MY STUDENTS SAY?

About Food and Drink: Melanie says,

"I drink a lot of water during days of training...When I eat right, I have more energy throughout the day, and during competitions, I have more power in stunting and tumbling."

About eating before performances, Kaitlyn says,

"We eat cliff bars before we perform. It helps sooooooo much. It gave us energy....if I don't eat before I practice or perform, I feel like I'm going to faint."

About Meals, Jade says,

"I eat three meals a day and several snacks."

About Performance, Anna says:

"Nutrition has affected my performance, because when I eat certain things, I just don't perform well."

About Junk Food, Lindsey says:

"If I ate a bunch of junk food, my muscles wouldn't be as strong."

About Endurance, Katie says:

"Nutrition makes a big difference on endurance and ability to practice for long periods of time...Also, in competitions, the less tired I am, the better I perform!"

TRANSITIONING

Keep in mind that changing over to a healthier diet does NOT have to be intense or drastic. Small changes make big differences, and you can work your way into the new diet. If you are a dedicated athlete and care about your body and health, don't delay.

The biggest thing is: Start Making a Change Today!

Transitioning to a better diet, you can start to substitute. Choose brown or wild rice or whole-wheat pasta in place of white rice and enriched flour ones. There are options of going gluten-free with pastas made from rice and corn flours. Replace your ordinary white sugar with pure cane sugar, agave nectar, or honey and table salt with sea salt. Start adding crunchy vegetables to replace chips.

Get your team together for morale support and make a plan. Talk to your parents and coach. Choose foods together.

Simple recipes like brown rice stuffing in baked green peppers or tomatoes and whole-wheat macaroni in macaroni & cheese makes your transitions easier. Make use of barley and bulgur wheat in mixed dishes, soup or stews and in casserole or stir-fries.

Start adding simple meats, chicken or fish with vegetables for dinner.

Drink vegetable heavy smoothies once daily, herbal teas, coconut water and water instead of carbonated drinks.

Substitute whole wheat or oat flour in pancake, waffle, muffin or other flour-based recipes with a bit more leavening for balance. Experiment with egg replacer and applesauce in place of eggs in certain baked pastries.

Let your imagination and nutritional education become your guide. If you are unfamiliar with some of these foods, be creative and investigate.

<u>Make it a fun adventure to a better you</u>!

GETTING STARTED?

First, you must make the <u>mental choice</u> that you will change and add these foods and schedules to your day. If this represents a big change in your life, break it down to something you can do. Say "I will try this new

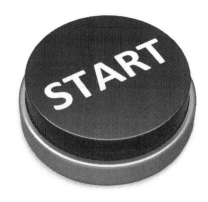

approach for <u>two weeks</u> and be dedicated to it, no matter what." Set your goal, and remember this is to be a better athlete and a better you. Are you serious about competing and being the best you can be? <u>Then commit</u>!

Next, make lists and write down ideas of what will be in your five or six small meals per day. Write down your typical meals and mealtimes on the left side of a paper, and the new meals and mealtimes on the right side of a paper. Make it clear in your head what you are doing. <u>Plan ahead</u>! Get your mom, your friends and teammates involved. Work together. Make it fun.

My daily ideal meal times

Meal 1:

Meal 2:

Meal 3:

Meal 4:

Meal 5:

Are you including more fruit, more vegetables, the kinds of foods I am recommending? Do you have those snacks and drinks ready to take to school each day, to keep your body hydrated and nourished? These lists and plans will help you with your grocery list.

HINT

Get your team together and designate an empty sports locker. Then fill it up with healthy snacks and fruits. Before, during and after practice you and your teammates can snack on the right foods, and have them easily accessible. Everyone gives $5 per week, for instance, and one student, coach or parent is in charge of replenishing the team nutrition locker from your list.

Good team snacks to keep handy and in my practice locker for teammates to stay properly fueled...

_____

_____

_____

_____

_____

_____

Next, when shopping at the grocery store (with your family or alone) for your personal meals, you should be looking for those foods that help to maximize your body's performance. With technology making research such a snap, look online for healthy recipes to know what ingredients to purchase. I include some in this book, too. But don't just familiarize yourself with what you buy. Also know the ingredients in each product.

Do not be fooled by foods labeled with the words "multi-grain," "stone-ground," "100% wheat," "cracked wheat," "seven-grain," or "bran." Frequently these may not be whole-grain products. Molasses or other additives can give what you think is a whole grain bread its brownish color. Read ingredient lists carefully to see if it is truly a whole grain food.

Look for terms that indicate added sugars (sucrose, high-fructose corn syrup, honey, and molasses) and oils (partially hydrogenated vegetable oils) to avoid those that add extra, usually empty calories. Instead pick those foods with fewer added sugars in whatever form.

Read labels carefully. This is essential, so commit to it. Since everything is about getting into a routine try it for two weeks or a month. Before you know it, it will become second nature. If you are too young to shop for yourself, talk with your parents and discuss how you can all eat better as a family. Positively influencing your household and those around you will result in healthy eating habits for you and those in your environment. It will also make it easier for you to fully embrace that healthier lifestyle.

An excellent website has tips for kids on reading labels and eating good foods. The link to reading labels is http://www.fda.gov/Food/ResourcesForYou/Consumers/NFLPM/default.htm

In order to reap the benefits of performing at a higher level of competition in cheerleading or any sport, your body demands that you must choose the right foods to fuel it.

MAKE OR BREAK YOUR GAME WITH THE FOOD YOU EAT!

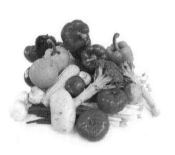

This might be a drastic change for some of you, but remember it is YOUR choice and the goal is worthy, which leads to the next rule:

RULE #7: I can become the best athlete I can with the ultimate competitive edge – making great daily choices!

These nutritional practices will become regular everyday habits, not just for event time. Condition the body to *always* be ready and in peak condition to be at your best at all times. Don't wait for the week before a competition to prepare yourself for the things you should have already had in action. Winners are always prepared for a win, at all costs.

Jade says: *"Nutrition makes a big difference. It gives me energy for games and competitions."*

Leanna says, *"Nutrition is very important because if you don't eat right you don't perform well, which I started realizing this year…it makes a huge difference in every way!"*

One more little tip: Enlist help from your doctor. Knowing your blood type will assist in determining your best diet. Different blood types require more or less of specific nutrients so having that information will help you to see what your body processes best. It will maximize how much energy can be built from what you eat. That information should be easily attainable from your medical records.

<u>Here are all of the Rules so far:</u>

▶ *RULE #1: It is absolutely necessary to take control of what I put into my body.*

▶ *RULE #2: I must be willing to make a change and new choices. I must be willing to break out of my old habits.*

▶ *RULE #3: Ideally, I will eat five times a day roughly totaling a 2,200 to 2,500 caloric intake. I can make or break my game with the food I eat!*

▶ *RULE #4: Eat well the night before and 3 hours before a practice or a competition to eliminate fatigue, lack of physical strength and undernourished muscles.*

▶ *RULE #5: After the hard work of a competition or workout, I will eat a small meal within thirty minutes of completion to replenish my muscles and energy stores (for better recovery.)*

▶ *RULE #6: Plan Ahead!*

▶ *RULE #7: I can become the best athlete I can with the ultimate competitive edge -- making great daily choices!*

"You will never "find" time for anything. If you want time, you must make it."

— CHARLES BRUXTON

CHAPTER 4

QUESTIONS & ANSWERS PLUS STORIES FROM GIRLS TODAY

Let me share some of the most frequent questions that my students and athletes ask, and this will help me explain information in more detail:

Q: WHY AM I ALWAYS FATIGUED BEFORE, DURING, AND AFTER PRACTICE?

Working in a female dominated sport, I see that appearance is everything -- and feelings of not being good enough, thin enough, etc. do creep in. There are so many fad diets out there which girls follow in their quest to get thinner. As we have learned, food is your fuel. If you follow fad diets, most will not supply

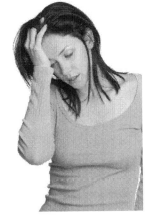

your body, muscles and tissues with what you need. You will end up being fatigued, or worse.

Feelings of fatigue prior to practice are usually because you are not fueling your body with the proper nutrients to support you in your sport. Any food or food combination that makes you sleepy thirty minutes later did not provide your body with the adequate nutrition required to perform at its max. Always pay attention to what your body is telling you. It will rarely be wrong.

Some coaches with less experience than me don't understand why I always require athletes to have a cliff bar/ protein bar/nut bar before practice - usually an hour before and one during practice. Athletes need to stay fueled throughout their practices.

Allow time at practices, such as a five minute "healthy snack break". Ask your coaches to build in this time, because some don't have a nutritional background: they will be more than willing to give up five minutes knowing they'll get better performances and results from their athletes. Please use that time to consume nutritionally sound snacks such as nuts, cliff bars, fruits, and juice or Gatorade. You can find more examples of healthy snacks in the food diary index.

I mentioned this earlier — I have found over time that athletes are less inclined to buy fast food after a practice or lesson if they had a protein bar snack and ate properly before practice or competition.

Muscles need carbohydrates. Along with dehydration, the lack of glycogen, supplied to the muscles through carbohydrates, is the most common factors contributing to an athlete's exhaustion.

Balanced diets high in carbohydrates have been proven to allow an athlete to significantly train or perform longer. Studies suggest that athletes insure they eat foods high in carbohydrates immediately after a practice or trial/game to provide the glucose needed after their stores in their muscle and liver have been tapped from exertion. However, avoid consuming any carbohydrates one and a half to two hours before an event. This may lead to premature exhaustion of glycogen stores in endurance events.

Q: WHAT ELSE DO I NEED TO AVOID FATIGUE AND KEEP PERFORMANCE UP? PROTEIN!

Dry beans and peas are part of both the protein and the vegetable groups. Animal sourced proteins (*red and white meats, poultry including eggs, seafood and dairy products*) are rich in essential amino acids. Soy, a common vegetable-based protein, is also a good source of essential amino acids. When consuming meat choose lean or low-fat options. Fish, nuts, and seeds contain healthy oils, so pick these foods frequently over other meats or poultry. Equipping your body with any or a combination of these protein sources before or after a workout will support muscle development and muscle repair.

Q: WHY CAN'T I INCREASE MY ENERGY WITH SUGAR?

Attempting to increase your energy by eating sugar or honey before an event does not work. In fact it may do just the opposite, with the 30 minutes it takes for the sugar to enter the blood stream. Because water is needed to absorb the sugar into the cells, this practice may also lead to dehydration. The surge of insulin it triggers causes a sharp drop in blood sugar level in those same 30 minutes. <u>Low blood sugar level leads to fatigue, nausea and dehydration.</u>

Q: WHAT ARE OTHER SECRETS TO HELP ME BEAT FATIGUE BEFORE COMPETITIONS OR PRACTICE?

Avoid meals high in fats, fiber and lactose (*dairy*). These foods take longer to digest than the nutrients found in fruits/vegetables. Furthermore, digestion time may pull away from your performance time.

Q: WHAT SHOULD I BE DOING TO INCREASE MY CALCIUM AND VITAMIN D INTAKE?

Calcium is an important component to anyone's well-being and is vital to bone health and muscle function. Female athletes in particular should have an ample supply of calcium to prevent the loss of that element that contributes to osteoporosis later on in life. Women are more likely to suffer from the disorder than men.

The best known sources of calcium are low-fat dairy products. If you are not a fan of or are intolerant to dairy products (*animal milk derived foods such as cheese, yogurt, ice cream, etc.*) try almond, rice, coconut, hemp, flaxseed or soy based milk products or vitamin supplements to help boost your system with these significant nutrients. Frequently these alternatives are fortified to have as much if not more calcium than its equivalent dairy counterpart without the mucus producing side-effects.

Somewhat less than 40% of people in the world retain the ability to digest lactose after childhood. The numbers are often given as close to 0% of Native Americans, 5% of Asians, 25% of African and Caribbean peoples, 50% of Mediterranean peoples and 90% of northern Europeans. Sweden has one of the world's highest percentages of "http://www.svenskmjolk.se/Templates/StartPage.aspx" Lactase tolerant people. (Weise, USAToday.com).[2]

Vegetables such as bok choy, broccoli, collards, Chinese cabbage, kale, mustard greens, and okra are excellent **natural sources of calcium** and are absorbed by the body easier. Reed Mangels, Ph.D., R.D. in the book, Simply Vegan: Quick Vegetarian Meals[3] reports that, "there is as much or more... calcium in ¾ cup of collard greens as there is in one cup of cow milk." So there is no reason that anyone cannot get the calcium they need.

You need vitamin D to absorb calcium. You cannot have one without the other. Fortified orange juice, cereals and milks are easy vitamin D sources. Likewise, the sun is the most natural source of vitamin D. It will benefit you to spend thirty minutes or more per day outside under the warm glow of our brightest star.

A final note about dairy comes from the International Sports Sciences Association. Frederick C. Hatfield PhD, author of Fitness: The Complete Guide [4] writes about a myth common among athletes concerning the formation of cellulite (*cottage cheese*) on thighs from consuming too much dairy It is just that - a myth. His research finds:

The activity of the fat promoting enzyme, lipoprotein lipase, is very high in the thighs and hips of women, resulting in a higher percentage of fat deposition in those areas. Women who have children need this accumulation to prepare for pregnancy and lactation. In addition the dimpling that is associated with cellulite is due to the deposit of fat and fibrous tissue. While an increase in overall body fat does play a role, it is also due to genetics. Deep massaging every night to break up the deposits of fat and fibrous tissue can help to temporarily decrease the appearance of the dimpling.

Q. HOW MUCH WATER SHOULD I DRINK BEFORE, DURING AND AFTER PRACTICE?

Water is unequivocally important to our diets. An average person can survive weeks, even months without eating but only about 3 days without water. Water is a must. It has the ability to move in and outside our cells transporting vital nutrients and other substances throughout the body that complete crucial metabolic and chemical reactions and handles cell maintenance. Water regulates your body's temperature, and maintains your body's structure and protection.

As mentioned earlier, we are composed of approximately 60-70% water. It is suggested that you drink half of your weight in ounces per day to maintain that balance. (*Your weight = 100lbs. You should be drinking at least 50 oz of water*). Interestingly we ingest most of our daily water through what we eat.

In addition to a surplus of essential vitamins and minerals, an apple is about 84% water, fresh broccoli 91%. A raw cucumber is a whopping 96% water. So it stands to reason if you are not getting your minimum amount of water per day to keep your own 60-70% in balance, increasing your consumption of fresh fruits and/or vegetables will definitely help. If you are not following a healthy diet, then drink more water (5).

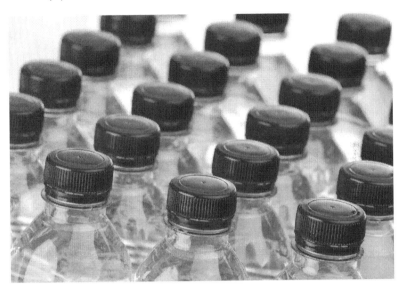

Lack of water can lead to dehydration which can be disastrous. Dehydrated muscles are prone to cramp and lock up. Outside of physical fatigue, your dehydrated brain cannot think and strategize clearly, a necessity for you as a serious athlete. Respiratory functions and heart rates can become challenged and the immune system becomes less effective. Though it is fairly easy to keep your body hydrated at any time, it can take up 36 hours to rehydrate your body once you have become dehydrated. So stay hydrated.

Katie says, "On training days, I drink three bottles of water and a bottle or two of Gatorade or coconut water."

Q: HOW MUCH WATER SHOULD I DRINK?

You must be consciously aware of your water intake regardless of thirst. Intense exercise can inhibit thirst, especially exercise lasting longer than an hour. **When possible, you should drink four ounces of water before practice and drink water every fifteen minutes throughout your practices to keep your body properly hydrated.** If you are not working out you should be drinking water at room temperature. It is recommended, by several credible sources, to drink mainly cold water during physical activities.

Water may not be quite enough because of the minerals we lose when we sweat, breathe or perform any other basic functions. It has been proven that we also lose sodium (*Na*), magnesium (*Mg*) and potassium (*K*), minerals often missing from plain tap water and needed for our body to maintain homeostasis. Human homeostasis is the body's ability to physically control its insides to ensure balance in response to changes outside. To this end, consider water that is <u>enhanced with electrolytes</u>, electrically-charged ions used to maintain voltages across cell membranes and carry electrical impulses across themselves and to other cells especially those of the nerve, heart and muscles.

<u>Simply put, electrolyte-enhanced water hydrates better than plain water because it replaces some of the critical minerals you lose while working out.</u> Coconut water is an excellent natural replenishing, mineral rich drink and is sold in single servings for the on-the-go athlete.

Although I am stressing the importance of fluids such as water, as with anything else in life, be sure to use moderation.

There is such a thing as drinking too much water. Ingesting too much of water before practice can lead to vomiting and even death.

Q: WHAT ABOUT CAFFEINE?

Water and liquids are obviously essential. Take in adequate fluids during pre-game time. However, avoid caffeine (*cola, coffee*) because it can lead to dehydration. Studies have shown that caffeine ingestion can indeed enhance endurance performance. However the beneficial effects of caffeine on performance are negated in people who use caffeine regularly. In other words caffeine can enhance aerobic performance for some but too much can be problematic. As I said earlier, 100% juices, smoothies and water will assimilate faster and give your body the hydration it will need and more healthy energy to run on.

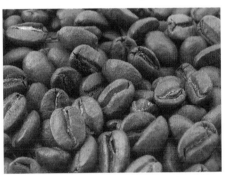

The energy of the food you put in your body is the energy you will get out, and this helps you avoid fatigue!

Q: WHY ARE SOFT DRINKS BAD FOR ME AS AN ATHLETE?

Do not attempt to substitute other drinks such as sodas and diet soda for your daily fluids. Contrary to popular belief, there is <u>nothing</u> healthy about diet sodas; colas in particular. As I have already said, consumption of soda leeches away important vitamins and minerals from your bones, leaving them weakened and with unhealthy growth.

They are, "...simply water with "http://www.diseaseproof.com/archives/diabetes-diet-drinks-for-preventing-diabetes-no-way.html" artificial sweeteners and other chemical additives, such as phosphoric acid"[5].

The safety of artificial sweeteners has been a "http://www.examiner.com/x-36995-Philadelphia-Family-Health-Examiner%7Ey2010m6d30-Are-artificial-sweeteners-effective-for-cutting-calories--Are-they-safe"[6] question of debate for years and their intense sweetness interrupts the body's natural association between, for instance, taste and nourishment, leading to weight gain. Phosphorus, the source of phosphoric acid is an important component in bone mineral but a high ratio of phosphorus to calcium can cause an event known to increase bone breakdown and decrease bone formation called parathyroid hormone secretion. Increasing your intake of calcium will not necessarily combat the effects that the increase of phosphorous on your bones. This is especially true and important for young women but does apply across gender lines. High phosphorus intakes acutely and negatively affect calcium and bone metabolism in a dose-dependent manner in healthy young females. This makes it very likely that the phosphorus content of colas generates calcium loss and that can lead to osteoporosis and bone degeneration. But that's not all!

These drinks are linked to "http://www.diseaseproof.com/archives/hurtful-food-sodium-and-artificial-sweeteners-linked-to-decline-in-kidney-function.html"[7] kidney dysfunction and advances obesity among other common medical problems.

Again, I know about this first hand. Though I am only 29 years old, I sometimes feel like I'm at least 65 years old. Do you know why? Because I ignored these facts as a child. Though my parents stressed the importance of avoiding soda, I consumed about 3-6 cans per day. I finally changed my habits and follow my own advice now, but I didn't when I was younger. Disobedience will catch-up to you.

...researchers discovered that parathyroid hormone (*PTH*) concentrations rise strongly following diet soda consumption. PTH functions to increase blood calcium concentrations by stimulating bone breakdown, and as a result release calcium from bone.

In the study, women aged 18-40 were given 24 ounces of either diet cola or water on two consecutive days, and urinary calcium content was measured for three hours. Women who drank diet cola did indeed excrete more calcium in their urine compared to women who drank water. The authors concluded that this calcium loss may underlie the observed connection between soda drinking and low bone mineral density.

Although caffeine is known to increase calcium excretion and promote bone loss, caffeine is likely not the only bone-harming ingredient in sodas. A 2006 study in the American Journal of Clinical Nutrition found consistent associations between low bone mineral density and caffeinated and non-caffeinated cola (*both regular and diet*), but not other carbonated beverages. One major difference between the two is the phosphoric acid in colas is absent from most other carbonated beverages.

In the Western diet, phosphorus is commonly consumed in excess – at about 3 times the recommended levels, whereas dietary "http://www.diseaseproof.com/archives/healthy-food-bok-choy-nutrient-dense-and-delicious.html"[8] calcium often low. Although phosphorus is an important component of bone mineral, a high dietary ratio of phosphorus to calcium can increase parathyroid hormone secretion, which is known to increase bone breakdown. Studies in which women were given increasing quantities of dietary phosphorus found increases in markers of bone breakdown and decreases in markers of bone formation. Therefore it is likely that the phosphorus content of colas, triggers calcium loss.

(NS Larson, et al "Effect of Diet Cola on urine calcium excretion" endojournals.org)

Q: HOW CAN I AVOID GETTING SICK DURING THE SEASON?

One of the most critical times for cheerleading comes in the late fall and early winter seasons. If you live in a state that is not warm during those times, cold and flu season will affect most of the members of your team at one time or another.

What if I told you there are easy ways to significantly reduce your team from getting sick?

Since we spend most of the year in close contact with the individuals on our teams we have to be mindful about sharing drinks and making sure we are eating the very best we can during cold season months. Falling sick not only affects your health but that of your teammates as well. Even if you don't infect others with your ailment, your absence compromises the integrity of your team.

RULE # 8: I WILL KEEP MY IMMUNE SYSTEM STRONG.

It is recommended that you consume chicken noodle soup *(avoid those with high sodium contents, artificial additives of sugar),* red peppers, oregano herb and oil, ginger and garlic to help keep your immune system strong. These will help you fight off cold and flu viruses. If you are following my recommendations, you are eating plenty of fresh fruits and vegetables which support the immune system, too. Fresh herbs, such as thyme, rosemary, parsley, cilantro, oregano, basil, dill, chives, and sage provide great health benefits to your body. These herbs are just as essential to your body in fighting off diseases and improving bodily functions as are vegetables and vitamins. Take an independent look at which herbs are good for what organs and ailments.

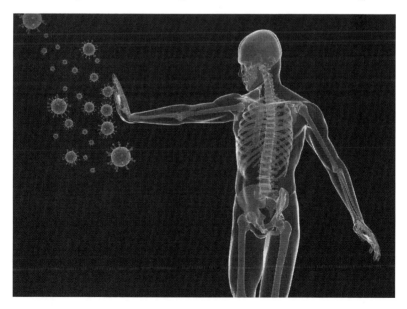

WINTER FRIENDLY FOODS:

During the winter months when the cold virus is looking for a home, consider these healthy options to keep your immunity system up and miss less practice.

Cayenne peppers	*improves blood circulation*
Celery	*immunity builder, potassium/sodium rich, etc.*
Dark, leafy vegetables such as kale	*calcium, vitamin K & B6, etc...*
collards	*copper, iron, vitamin C, etc...*
broccoli	*cancer fighter, potassium, vitamin A, etc...*
Brussels sprouts	*folic acid, beta carotene, etc...*
Chips and salsa	*Easily made at home with chopped tomatoes [or sub red bell peppers], cilantro, garlic and onions with a fresh squeeze of lime*
Elderberry	*immune booster, antiviral, antioxidant*
Fortified orange juice	calcium and vitamin C

Garlic	*antibacterial, antibiotic*
Ginger	*immune booster, anti-inflammatory, etc. - buy it fresh.* 1. Chop it up and pour on hot water for a tea option 2. Thinly sliced it into a stir-fry 3. Juice it and add it to your smoothies.)
Medicinal mushrooms	*calcium, iron, antibacterial, anti-inflammatory, antiviral, etc.* Shiitake, maitake, reishi, and more!
Red peppers	*a great ally against your teammates' flu*
Turmeric	*antibacterial, antioxidant*

Increase your supplement intake during these months with Echinacea, vitamin D3, zinc, selenium, and probiotics. Incorporate aloe vera juice in your smoothies and teas.

Always drink plenty of fluids and get adequate rest to support your immune system. Add soy to your diet. It has been shown by researchers that people who consume soy protein and isoflavones are leaner and less likely to become overweight – and most people put on weight during the winter.

Know the truth about foods - to keep your body and your immune system strong!

Education in nutrition needs to be practical, to address eating strategies and key food and fluid choices and achieve the goals of sound nutrition. Knowing exactly what you are eating is the best way to take over your diet.

My weekly detailed food intake

....

....

....

....

....

....

....

....

....

....

....

....

....

....

....

....

....

....

....

....

....

....

....

....

....

Again, you don't have to give up all of your favorite foods. That would be impractical - but you can begin by compensating your guilty pleasures for healthier versions. Make small changes from sodas to natural juices, fried foods to baked ones, white bread to whole wheat bread (*leave the crust on - it's okay*) and from table salt to sea salt.

We learned earlier that medical studies say soft drinks do you more harm than good, and that fast foods eat away at your energy rather than adding to it. If what you eat and drink makes you sleepy, that meal has depressed your body's system and didn't do its job properly, thereby preventing you from doing your job properly. Food should give you energy, not take it away. If you find this to be the case with a certain food or drink, immediately reduce its place in your diet.

Take for example a high fat meal, one consisting of fried, fatty, high sodium, processed meats, white bread that is essentially wheat bread with all of the vital nutrients and enzymes removed, and some sugary dessert or drink to finish it off; in other words your basic fast food restaurant combo.

On average the meat portions of the above meal are full of saturated fats which are widely known to raise LDL (*low-density lipoprotein*) cholesterol levels, known as the "bad" cholesterol in people, which in turn raises the chances for heart disease, strokes and certain kinds of cancer. Add to that, many of those fats are also trans fats which are known to decrease one's good HDL (*high-density lipoprotein*) cholesterol, thereby boosting one's potential for type 2 diabetes and both colon and breast cancer.

These high fat, nutritionally stripped and depleted foods digest more slowly, leading to the fatigue associated with poor diet. Add processed white sugar to the combo via a dessert or soda and now you have a spike in blood sugar which gives a very temporary energy boost while releasing insulin into the body, allowing the body to more easily store fat. The sharp decline in blood sugar that follows makes for even less energy. Next, those same sweets can draw hydrating fluids into the gastrointestinal tract, away from where they are otherwise needed and lead to dehydration, cramps and nausea. <u>All of this from one average fast food meal</u>. Not exactly the lifestyle any athlete wants to lead.

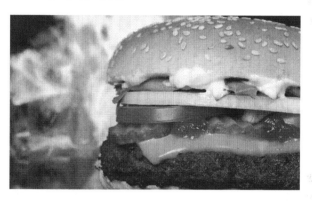

YOU HAVE A CHOICE:

Live a long, comfortable and healthy life by educating yourself on the foods
you eat every day and exercising that knowledge with delicious and nourishing choice at your table

OR

Live a life ingesting numerous prescription medicines with varying side effects, poor health, in need of assistance and continuous trips to the hospital.

Q: SO, ARE YOU SAYING THAT EATING POORLY CAN ACTUALLY CAUSE DISEASES?

Yes. Living a healthier lifestyle results in you feeling better and decreases the risk of serious nutrient-deficient based diseases. When you eat well, you feel great and it's not a feeling that comes and goes. It's a feeling that stays and allows you to be productive and more adventurous with a reduced risk of diseases. When you feel good as an athlete, you can perform and compete better.

> Nutritional intake has proven to be one of the most important factors with regard to the prevention and treatment of these diseases. The influence of nutrition can be both a matter of what is eaten that supports the development of these diseases or supports the prevention or slows the progression of these diseases. Heart disease and cancer account for more than 60 percent of deaths in the US.[vi]

You have to become responsible for your body and well-being. Your willingness to educate yourself and be conscientiously aware of what you are eating can make that process fun and easy. You can do it!

Q: I HEAR ABOUT SODIUM IN OUR DIET. IS IT BAD?

Sodium is not good for you and can cause high blood pressure among other things. Most sodium in the food supply comes from packaged foods. Similarly packaged foods can differ greatly in sodium content, including breads. Use the "http://www.choosemyplate.gov/food-groups/downloads/TenTips/DGTipsheet14SaltAndSodium.pdf "http://www.mypyramid.

68

gov / related_links / index.html" \ l "nutritionfacts" Nutrition Facts" label, found on most food packaging in the U.S., to choose foods with a lower % DV for sodium.

Foods with less than 140 mg sodium per serving can be labeled as low sodium foods. Claims such as "low in sodium" or "very low in sodium" on the front of the food label can help you identify foods that contain less salt (or sodium).

Processed meats such as ham, sausage, hotdogs, and luncheon/deli meats can have a surplus of added sodium. Most fresh meats in your average grocery store have been enhanced with a salt-containing solution adding significant amounts of sodium. Check the " "http://www.mypyramid. gov / related_links / index.html" \ l "nutritionfacts" Nutrition Facts" label to know what kind of sodium intake you will be eating in that particular food product. Scan the product label for wording such as "self-basting" or "contains up to __% of __", which mean that a sodium-containing solution is in that product.

Most oils are high in mono or polyunsaturated fats and low in saturated fats. Oils from plant sources (vegetable and nut oils) do not contain any cholesterol. In fact, no foods from plants sources contain cholesterol.

A few plant oils, however, including coconut oil and palm kernel oil, are high in saturated fats and for nutritional purposes are considered to be "http://www.mypyramid.gov/ pyramid/discretionary_calories_fats.html" solid fats. Solid fats are fats that are solid at room temperature, like butter and shortening. Solid fats come from many animal foods and can be made from vegetable oils through a process called hydrogenation.

Some common solid fats are:

- butter

- beef fat (*tallow, suet*)

- chicken fat

- pork fat (*lard*)

- stick margarine

- shortening

Limit, if not completely eliminate these fats from your diet. The same way these oils congeal (*the process of going from their heated liquid state to their cooled solid state*) when sitting out is the same thing it does in your body, clogging up your insides. Yuk! Our average 98.6° body temperature is well below what it takes to change those oils back into their liquid form for easy digestion.

BE THE BEST YOU CAN BE – INSIDE AND OUT!

Q: WHAT ABOUT MY DOWNTIME ROUTINE?

I will repeat this - condition your body to *always* be ready and in peak condition to be at your best. Don't wait for the week before a competition to eat better. Prepare yourself for the things you should have already had in action.

In your downtime if you find yourself at home, eating unhealthy foods and watching television on the couch or in your bed, you will consequently find something not right with your body. You will feel tired and not look very good. That is your body talking to you – and you should listen.

Consider becoming more active by changing not only your eating habits during training and performance time, but your habits all the time. Call it your lifestyle choice! With that in mind, find constructive things to do on your downtime instead of becoming a couch potato.

If you have access to a treadmill, walk on it three to four times daily while reading your favorite book. Or do a fast paced walk for four minutes followed by a fast sprint run for two minutes while listening to some new music. Play sports, ride a bike, play tennis, do activities that you like and have fun.

If none of these options appeal to you, try moving yourself from the couch to the floor to stretch while watching TV or doing homework. Do some yoga, or have a jump rope or light weights you can use during TV commercials or when you need a break from your homework. This will cause you to burn calories, while simultaneously working your mind and body.

RULE #9: I will have fun! I won't ignore the psychological aspect of fun while choosing discipline in my life. I can attain peak performance as an athlete!

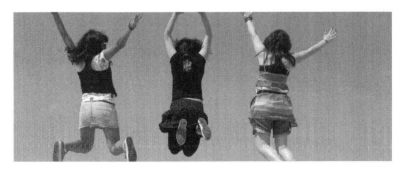

"The will to win means nothing without the will to prepare."

—JUMA IKANGAA
(OLYMPIC MARATHON RUNNER)

CHAPTER 5

EXERCISE AND BODY MOVEMENT "PRACTICE MAKES PERFECT!"

Disclaimer: *Before doing any of these exercises or participating in any physical exercise program or diet, make sure to consult your physician or personal trainer.*

As an immigrant child who came to America at the age of nine, my world view is going to be a bit different from many others.

For me, being in America gave me the chance to play and excel at sports, something girls didn't do in Haiti. At first, I weighed only about 66 pounds and had no real muscle structure. I'm sure I looked like one of the kids on a UNICEF commercial asking for financial support to be fed and kept alive!

After being in the country for about a year, I started to play many sports. Unfortunately I had no real passion. I was great at all of them. My sports included cross country, and I broke the school record for the mile run. I did track, played volleyball and then gymnastics, where I begin to feel a connection to my sport. I was a natural tumbler and able to execute difficult and new skills instantly.

As I continued to excel in tumbling, I started going to the gym daily and watch college and club gymnastics to understand where I needed to reach. After two years of consistently gaining skills, my older sister, also in gymnastics, got injured and since she was the primary reason I tried gymnastics in the first place, I looked for another option that seemed less dangerous. I found cheerleading since it had the basic elements of gymnastics and was heavily based on tumbling. I was a great asset to my Junior High squad, since I was the only person that came from a gymnastics background and could tumble.

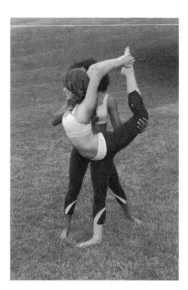

A common notion among cheerleading illiterates is that it is not a real sport. In order for this perception to change, we must consistently display our athleticism and sportsmanlike conduct. We can achieve this level of greatness by being completely dedicated to our work, both in and out of practice.

I instruct more than 40 hours of private lessons per week. Having taught tumbling now for many years, I have worked with and built a good share of great athletes. What do I know from observing student athletes over the years? **The best** are those that make the most out of their time inside and outside the gym, and choose discipline and dedication!

While researching for this book I came across a concept that I strongly believe and pass on to my athletes. It's the most valid concept that I have read so far and is a great rule for all athletes to live by:

The Rule of 10,000

In his book, <u>Outliers: The Story of Success</u>, author Malcolm Gladwell who made the reference based on the research by Anders Ericsson says that he discovered the key to success in *any* field – and he studied and observed many highly successful people including athletes. <u>Experts who have practiced at their skill for at least 10,000 hours attain superior success</u>. This includes competitive cheerleaders in college and professional sports cheerleading teams. This takes us to the next rule.

RULE #10: Practice, Practice, Practice!

One must become a polished performer to advance amidst the changing dynamics of cheering. The cheerleader's skills are pushed to the limit on a daily basis. It is all about *Practice, Practice, Practice!* This goes for every athlete and every sport.

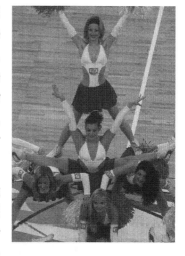

I make sure that my tumbling students practice their turns and increase to at least 4 turns per minute. In practice or at camp

I increase the repetitions of the taught skills. For instance, during Katie's private lessons she tumbles about 5 times per minute which then becomes over 250 turns per hour lesson - with about ten minutes for water breaks and snack time. If your household is investing in private lessons and you're not tumbling at least 100 times in an hour, chances are you're not going to successfully master any new skills or the confidence in the current skills. You aren't applying enough time to the skill. Not mastering a skill can lead to mental blocks and decreased confidence. That is bad for all parties involved. This leads us to the next rule.

RULE #11: It is important to challenge myself and be fully immersed in whatever I do to be the best.

SOME PERSONAL OBSERVATIONS

To stay immersed in this field, I am an official cheerleading judge for Illinois high schools governing body. So, throughout the competitive season, I get to judge a large number of teams based on established and known rubrics.

I observe that some athletes put in extra time to research and understand what cheerleading, or their particular sport, is all about. When I was a high school cheerleader I would look to Allstar and collegiate programs for inspiration. Nowadays the best places to look are competitive cheerleading and college cheerleading. You can buy nationals videos online without having any affiliations. You can seek out YouTube videos. You can find information on the internet. Some cheerleaders have no idea what the sport is about or what it entails. Now it's time to find out how to maximize your skills.

This leads to the next rule.

Rule #12: I will do my research and stay current with rules, trends and competitive moves!

The better prepared you are for potential challenges the more success you will have in ANY sport. Go online to sites like YouTube to study cheering routines, the latest swim meet rules, gymnastic advances, track and field rules. Bone up on the latest soccer or volleyball moves. Attend local competitions to see what other teams or athletes are doing. This will also ensure that you stay current with new rules and trends – and it will help guarantee you a longer career with fewer injuries.

LACK OF PREPARATION

One of the most irritating issues I run across when coaching is an athlete's lack of preparation. You should not assume you have good enough skills and therefore need to stop trying to improve them. Practice your motions and other basic skills with teammates and whatever else your coaches suggest can be improved.

I always advise cheerleading athletes to spend at least 20 minutes each day practicing on their own. Go through sidelines, cheers, routines, dances, motions, jumps and facials - all in front of a mirror. Practicing in front of a mirror will allow you to see what areas need improvement. The more you practice, the better you get. Why 20 minutes? For no other reason but to protect the vast amount of time and money you invest to master this sport.

WHAT ARE SOME AREAS OF PRACTICE THAT ARE IMPORTANT? WHAT SHOULD I BE DOING?

Conditioning and Stretching One of the best athletes that I have instructed in and out of practice will testify that she is always pushed to the limit to work as hard as she possibly can each day. Even when Katie is having an off day, she conditions and deep stretches.

As a coach to hundreds of athletes, <u>I find that there are two types of athletes: those who work hard and those who hardly work.</u>

Listen, why go through the trouble of devoting yourself to a sport only to slack and not give it your best? Being lazy and apathetic toward your sport is not wise and can even be perilous. I unfortunately come across lazy athletes more often than I would like. In such instances, it poses a serious challenge to me as a coach to find creative ways to motivate to change their behavior and advance individually and better perform for their programs.

What can you do to challenge yourself today? This is a basic question I often ask athletes. So, why don't you list three things you can do to challenge yourself more this week:

1. _____

2. _____

3. _____

PROTECT YOUR BODY

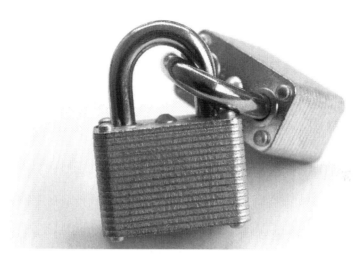

Since cheerleading is such a dangerous sport, you *must* condition and stretch to avoid pulling muscles or breaking body parts. This requires daily time and effort and is to protect your body.

So look at it like this: When you study for a test, you go into the exam more secure in your ability to pass the test. But when you don't study at all, you go into the exam nervous and ill prepared, sure of the inevitability of receiving a bad grade. Well, the same concept applies to getting ready for a competition.

> *Kaitlyn says, "I typically practice 10 hours a week, though during football season it is 6 ½ hours (because of all the game time performing), but during competition period it can be 14 hours a week."*

> *Melanie says, "Athletes can improve their performance by practicing simple skills and working out every day."*

Brianna says, "In cheerleading, it is a never-ending cycle of having to learn new things to perfect. We can improve by conditioning, eating right and getting plenty of sleep!"

As a cheerleader, much like a student taking a test, there are expectations to do your homework and study so that your squad can excel on that 2:30-3:00 minute exam at the end of your competition season. The concept applies to all athletes.

Your <u>sports homework</u> might include this list:

- taking care of yourself

- regulating what and when you eat

- giving your all in practice

- conditioning and stretching outside of practice

- researching routines or rules

I am a strong believer in the idea that we make time for what we want to make time for. If I love watching my favorite television program I will make time to watch it, no matter what. The same consideration should be given when it comes to doing your sport homework.

I CANNOT STRESS THIS ENOUGH: STRETCH DAILY.

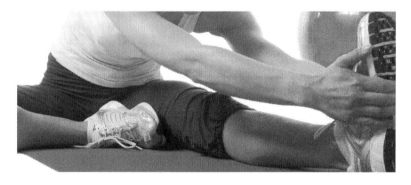

Stretching practices

Stretching enhances everything in any sport. In cheerleading, bases should be flexible as cheerleading includes extensive jumping and tumbling. If you are a flyer, then you absolutely need to know how to pull every body position. However strength and flexibility training must occur at the same time.

While coaches, including myself, emphasize the importance of *flexibility* for this sport, I also always inform my students of the importance of *strengthening* focused areas as well.

So while I encourage my students to stretch their splits daily for three minutes on each side, I also give them strengthening exercises for their hips and knees to maintain balance and physically increase their overall strength. This can help a cheerleader to excel faster and to safely demonstrate their skills.

Have a trainer or other professional teach you proper strengthening and stretching techniques to avoid injury or overexertion that you can do on your own. Not having all three splits can be detrimental.

As a base and a flyer, I regularly did straddle wall sits and splits on all three sides. I practiced my body positions on a chair, stair, or even a can of food. It was perpetual practice that made me proficiently flexible, not just natural ability.

Dedicating your time to stretching does work. Whether you are a base or a flyer, don't limit your flexibility potential. For those who have poor flexibility, simply push past the pain and stretch more frequently. This is definitely a rule!

Rule #13: Stretch, Stretch, Stretch!

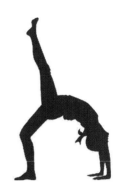

Some girls ask if their muscles will turn to fat if they stop exercising regularly. Let's put that fear to rest! Frederick C. Hatfield PhD, of the International Sports Sciences Association notes that "muscle and fat are two separate and distinct tissues on your body." That, "...muscles cannot turn into fat. They simply do not have the physical capability to change from one type of tissue to another. In reality, muscles have the unique property of "use it or lose it." If you do not use a muscle it will literally waste away (atrophy)" is what my doctor always tells me.

IS PRACTICE ENOUGH?

No, practice is not enough!

One of the most talented teams my company, Cheer Tumbling Dynamics, has ever worked with got a great routine from one of our best choreographers. Two weeks after completing their routine, I came back for a follow up visit to find not one athlete could recall what was taught in its entirety. If they went home and practiced their parts even eight times in the two week period, this would not have been an issue. <u>I knew that poor practice patterns led them down this road</u>. I had to explain to them, that they and not their coaches were accountable for memorizing their routines that they paid thousands of dollars for. If you don't practice outside of the hours handed to you by your coaches, chances are your performance will not improve.

Again, practice is not enough - that is, if you aspire to be the best and to excel.

Be prepared to dedicate more time to your sport. Each passing moment is time that could be spent improving your skills. To better prepare my lessons for learning and maintaining difficult skills, I assign daily conditioning exercises. It typically varies for each lesson based on the team's current condition of muscles and the future goals. This list gets adjusted monthly as skills improve and body types change.

I have provided you with a basic conditioning sample plan to keep you working on your muscles. This will help you to become proficient faster and to perform with better technique.

Do these exercises at your discretion and based on your physical and mental ability. I recommend that you mix and match these various exercises and change them up every week for greater variety.

DAILY CONDITIONING

Stretch your splits

Daily for three minutes on each side (*left, right and middle*).

HIP FLEXORS

30 lifts each side and the middle, with knees locked out and toes pointed. Sit in a straddle position, and pull one leg at a time, locked and pointed towards your face, and hold for one minute each.

4X8 PUSH-UP SET

Do 8 regular pushups, and then bend left leg up to your right knee. Do eight more pushups in this position and switch sides. Complete another set of eight then hold a plank (*arms straight, hands under shoulders in a locked position*) for 8 counts. Repeat this exercise 4 times.

4X30 LEG KICK 'N SQUATS

Put your feet together and kick one leg at a time in front of you and go into a low squat in between each kick.

60X2 CONTINUOUS LUNGES

Get in lunge position, pump in that position for 60 counts and switch sides.

50 TUCK ROLLS AND LAYOUT ROCKS

These should be done lying flat on your back, holding on to something stable like couch legs or the foot of a bed. Maintain a tight body position and lift both legs off the ground a little bit and roll up, with your toes up and knees coming towards the object that you're holding. Layout rock is your basic hollow body position and rocking on your bottom and lower back while squeezing your tummy and bottom as tight as you can.

4X50 LEG EXERCISES

50 paddles, 50 crisscross, 50 lifts, and 50 straddles. Keep hands under your butt.

50X3 CALF LIFTS

Calf lifts should be done for each leg, individually and then together.

4X8 CRUNCH SET

Doing crunches with different leg variations. Left, right, together, straddle. Repeat 4 times.

These exercises are beneficial to you, easy to do outside of the gym and are really important for your body. The better shape that you're in, the better your tumbling and other skills will grow. You can go on my website to see sample video exercises to help maintain better msucle strength. www.cheertd.com

SHOULD I LEARN TUMBLING FIRST?

In cheerleading, some girls ask me if they should learn tumbling before moving to cheer.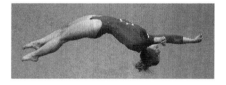

Tumbling constitutes 20% of most competitive score sheets, making it a big part of competitive cheerleading. It is abundantly advantageous to acquire at least basic tumbling skills. The more tumbling skills you possess, the more likely you will secure your place on a competitive or champion team. Most schools strive to have their entire squad tumbling to maximize score sheets. Maximize your full potential before pursuing a competitive squad.

If you are new to the sport, invest time learning your tumbling basics; handstands, cartwheels, round-offs, back and front walkovers, and back-handsprings. Getting those fundamentals down will give you a great starting point and a good means to move forward.

85

Tumble hard, courageous and smart!

Most sports require participants to display their physical athleticism, endurance and stamina. Cheerleading is no different. Strength and flexibility, therefore, has to be a standard within our cheerleading community. Important skills include: body strength through practice; better eating habits; stretching; and tumbling skills.

The earlier you begin tumbling, the better you will be in cheerleading. All tumbling skills require that you be in the *best* possible shape regarding your body size and strength. This can significantly reduce the risk of injury among athletes.

In an attempt to better display the required skills, there are always things you can do at home, in classes and before or after practice to improve your tumbling skills. You should be able to do handstand pushups against a wall or hold a handstand on your own. You should be able to hold your body in push up position for more than 20 seconds.

Be skeptical of tumbling coaches that lure you into lessons without the proper tumbling background. Ask for references and for phone numbers of past students. Inquire about the quality of their services, including any certifications or awards they may have earned. The easiest way to acquire a reputable coach is from the recommendation of family or friends or by simply calling your local gym and then doing your own research. Research sports facilities that offer cheerleading or gymnastics or both. Ask the owner for recommendations for distinguished coaches.

DO YOU LOVE BEING AN ATHLETE AND COMPETITOR?

If you love being an athlete and are dedicated to improving your skills, then get to work and you will see faster, stronger results!

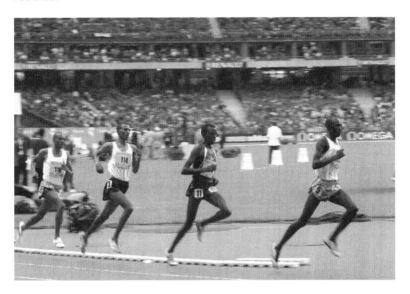

Here is a summary of the Rules in this Chapter:

▶ *RULE #10: Practice, Practice, Practice!*

▶ *RULE #11: It is important to challenge myself and be fully immersed in whatever I do to be the best.*

▶ *Rule #12: I will do my research and stay current with rules, trends and competitive moves!*

▶ *Rule #13: Stretch, Stretch, Stretch!*

"When you have developed motivation, discipline, and emotional control, becoming successful is a simple byproduct of this combination."
— VINCE LOMBARDI

CHAPTER **6**

ATTITUDE AND INNER STRENGTH "BE THE BEST YOU CAN BE!"

In this chapter, I share different observations and ideas to motivate you and let you in on some secrets. You have so much potential inside of you, and you can release it and soar!

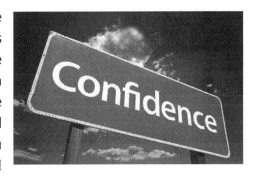

As much as practicing and eating right are important, even more important is your attitude and inner strength! It is your thoughts and belief in yourself that bring you to the next level. That is a secret to being the best you can be.

There are many inspirational leaders, whether they are athletes, inventors, politicians, musicians, etc. Leaders evolve in all fields. And they all have some similarities:

- They believe in themselves.

- They don't listen to the naysayers or people who don't believe in them.

- They are devoted to their field, apply themselves all the time (remember the Rule of 10,000?).

- They often inspire others through their dedication.

- If an athlete, they work to make their body the best it can be to support the mental "can-do" attitude.

- They have all failed at some time, but tried again (and again.)

These are all things you can do!

I have included a few more inspiration quotes from well know figures that may help inspire you:

"I've always believed that if you put in the work, the results will come. I don't do things half-heartedly. Because I know if I do, then I can expect half-hearted results."

– MICHAEL JORDAN

"Any reward that is worth having only comes to the industrious. The success which is made in any walk of life is measured almost exactly by the amount of hard work that is put into it."

– CALVIN COOLIDGE, US PRESIDENT

"The greatest force in our lives is our attitude. It's a power that is yours to define. If you decide it will be positive, you increase your personal power exponentially."
— COACH PAT RILEY

"Your life - the way it looks today is a result of your choices...What will you choose today for your tomorrows?"
— ROBERT G. ALLEN

"Don't let the noise of other's opinions drown out your own inner voice. And most important, have the courage to follow your heart and intuition."
—STEVE JOBS

"Somewhere behind the athlete you've become and the hours of practice and the coaches who have pushed you is a little girl who fell in love with the game and never looked back... play for her."
— MIA HAMM

"Start by doing what's necessary, then what's possible, and suddenly you are doing the impossible."
-FRANCIS OF ASSISI

"Ask not what your teammates can do for you. Ask what you can do for your teammates."
-MAGIC JOHNSON

"I really believe the only way to stay healthy is to eat properly, get your rest and exercise. If you don't exercise and do the other two, I still don't think it's going to help you that much."

— MIKE DITKA

"Success is measured by your discipline and inner peace."

— MIKE DITKA

"I always felt that my greatest asset was not my physical ability, it was my mental ability."

— BRUCE JENNER , GOLD MEDAL OLYMPICS

"Clear your mind of can't ".

— SAMUEL JOHNSON

"Energy and persistence conquer all things."

— BENJAMIN FRANKLIN

"Nothing can stop the man with the right mental attitude from achieving his goal; nothing on earth can help the man with the wrong mental attitude."

— THOMAS JEFFERSON

"Go confidently in the direction of your dreams. Live the life you have imagined.

— HENRY DAVID THOREAU

SUMMING UP SOME IMPORTANT POINTS

To be the best you can be, there are a few basic ideas I have discussed in the book – and a few more to add. Let's sum them up.

Discipline: discipline to take on new eating habits and stick to it, discipline to practice often and regularly, discipline to stretch often, discipline to research and learn more about your sport. A top competitor and champion has discipline.

I have added Joy, Inner Peace, Respect and Leadership to the list!

Joy: If you enjoy your sport and the camaraderie with your teammates, and if you enjoy the strength your body feels from good eating habits, you will feel happy and joyful. Even when you are still reaching for your goals; even if you lose a competition. You will feel motivated to be even better if you can harness these feelings. And it will show when you compete!

Inner Peace: This is sometimes hard to achieve. You are so busy with school, tests, exams, practices, dedication to tumbling and cheer, your families, other interests...sometimes it seems like there are not enough hours in the day and you are frazzled. However, by planning your days, taking control and also believing in yourself, you can calm some of the craziness. I like to take deep breaths with my eyes closed (like meditation) if even for a few minutes per day, to help calm myself. I do know from experience that if you are disciplined, this can bring inner peace. And then you are a better competitor and a better person!

Respect: Respect means respecting your body and your time, respecting your teammates, respecting your coaches, and even respecting your competition!

Leadership: Leaders go above and beyond, they inspire others, and help lead others to higher goals. Others look to leaders and want to be like them.

This all takes an investment of time and money

By now you should have realized that this is a very expensive sport especially since team practices are not enough to stay at the top. You'll invest in private tumbling lessons, flyer stretcher classes, flying classes, conditioning classes and more. To maximize your investment and minimize those costs consider what you can do additionally to enhance your skills and become a better cheerleader, such as the daily workout outlined earlier. Don't hesitate to ask your coaches what else you can do on your own to improve your skills.

Attitude: If you have a choreographer every year, please mimic them *exactly* before adding your own style or changes. Practice your motions in front of a mirror. Ask someone you look up to who has more cheerleading knowledge than you do, like your coach, or captain to assist you. Why? You are investing money and time into your sport, and you want to take the knowledge and experience from a choreographer to make you better. If you can grasp the work and research they are offering, and then practice this in front of a mirror and with more experienced people, it will help you improve and soar.

No matter how talented and skilled you are, don't let a bad attitude seep in. There is always someone more knowledgeable there to help you. Listen and incorporate ideas. Keep an open mind and positive attitude!

Knowledge is Power: We are living in a time where social media rules. <u>Use these tools to your advantage</u>. Look up national champions online, and read the various cheerleading magazines publications. Seek out your camp counselor for sound advice. There are even conferences for coaches to learn about the sport, rubrics and trends that will help your team. Find all resources, use them. Knowledge is power!

WHAT MAKES A GREAT LEADER?

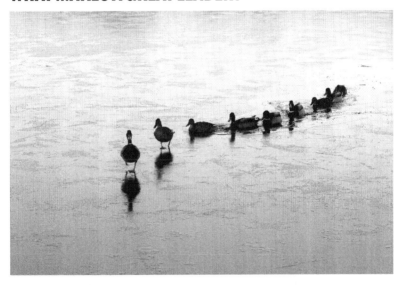

A great leader is one who goes above and beyond what is expected of them. They know how to lead and when to follow; will know how to take and give direction. One of my favorite songs, "Unwritten," by Natasha Beddingfield, illustrates this:

No one else can feel it for you
Only you can let it in...
no one else can speak the words on your lips...
Livin' your life with arms wide open
Today is where your book begins

It says that our futures are unwritten so we should stop setting limitations for ourselves or predicting what can and will happen. This is good advice and leads to our final rule:

RULE #12: I WILL MAKE MYSELF LIMITLESS!

With a little hard work you can create a great story about purpose, hard work, and success for yourself and your team. No one but *you* can determine what your future holds. Anything and everything is possible!

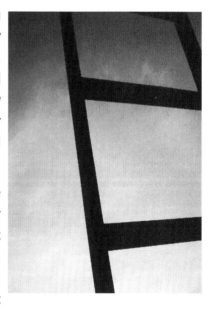

When my athletes are struggling with a new or difficult skill, the most common thing I hear from them is, "*I can't do it.*" I respond, "Then you won't do it," and say nothing else. The only way that we *can't* do something is if there is a physical or mental disability that hinders us. Aside from that and sometime, even despite those conditions, we *can do anything*. That's why you can go from having trouble throwing your tumbling or stunting skill one day then doing it perfectly the next. You simply choose to. You have the mental capacity. Once you decide to push yourself physically to practice consistently, you can overcome it.

When I was a high school cheerleader, I was the unofficial tumbling instructor for my coed cheer team. Our team was comprised of some big guys. I would teach them back handsprings, back tucks, round off back handsprings and other skills.

Ken, one of my best friends and a fellow captain, had a great round off back handspring that he was afraid to throw without having me spot him. Each day for a month, he left practice disappointed that he didn't give it his all because of his fear to flip backwards on his own, frustrating both himself and our coaches.

One day at the end of practice I advised Ken to have a conversation with himself when he was alone for the rest of the week. *I told him to see himself doing it over and over in his head and to talk himself up to it.*

Per this advice, the following week he came in and <u>executed the moves all by himself</u> despite my coaches' doubt. I think that perhaps that was a great moment in his life and mine as well. **It will be a great and defining moment in your life too when you push yourself further than anyone predicts.**

What I have observed after teaching for many years is that people can be quick to sell you short. This can be the cause of many of our fears and the source of our doubt in our own abilities. You can achieve anything you want in a sport like cheerleading. <u>The possibilities are endless because you determine your own progress and success by taking matters into your own hands.</u>

A great athlete does not play their sport solely with his/ her mind but with his/her heart as well. Hesitation will hinder you.

Tumble and Cheer with your heart, instinct, and physical ability!

Motivational cheerleading Motivational cheerleading represents millions of athletes in the United States. We are known to be trendsetters. We are among the leaders in our respective communities. Being a part of this respected sport gives us the opportunity to positively influence those around us. It is a great responsibility.

List here three things that you can do to develop a better attitude, to become a better leader to be more inspired:

1. _____

2. _____

3. _____

We must commit to learning the necessary skill sets to honor that responsibility. However, some athletes find themselves in a school environment that does not offer much respect to our sport. In such cases, it is simply a matter of leaning on the respect you have for yourself and cheering, which will then propel a similar respect from your peers.

And here are some final words:

Don't...

Don't ever let anyone tell you that you can't attain a skill.

Don't ever say "never." When you say that you can't, you won't.

Don't ever doubt yourself. **Confidence** *has a correlation with* **greatness.**

Don't ever allow a practice go to waste.

Don't come to your practices or to a competition without being mentally prepared.

Don't be overly analytical. You can become your own worst enemy.

Don't be a sore loser.

Don't put others down. It makes people question your character.

Don't quit in the middle of the season. It's not fair to the other people who worked hard with you all year. They shouldn't have to start over because of you.

Do...

Do keep up your grades.

Do look for encouragement in yourself before you do in others.

Do love and respect yourself so you can respect others.

Do try your hardest.

Do the most you can each practice.

Do encourage others to push themselves.

Do concentrate on your games and competitions enough to learn all aspects of the sport.

Do watch yourself practice motions in front of the mirror.

Do openly accept constructive criticism. Teammates are there to help you.

Do trust your coaches.

Do believe in yourself.

Do smile! You'll be surprised how much that can lift your spirits.

Let's end the book with advice from my own current and former athletes, speaking directly to you!

Corinne Piazza - *Live in the now and never get discouraged when you don't get what you want the first time.*

Amy Papesh - *You can never give up. When you really want something (a skill for example) you have to fight for that skill because it won't just be handed to you. It takes time.*

Sara-Anne Oberkirch – *The best way to improve is to change your mindset. Athletes need to have their heads in the game or else all of the nutrition and training in the world won't help!*

Anna Balinski – *I am motivated by the thought of getting better and stronger every day.*

Katie Oberkirsh - *I would say never give up. Always chase your dream and always stay positive, because a team is only as weak as its weakest person.*

Cricket Bishop - *Don't anticipate; participate.*

Katie Schelli – *Practice! But practice isn't effective without a healthy diet.*

Anisha Clay - *You definitely need practice. Stretch. Give every practice your all and support your team in order to succeed. Fearlessness helps too.*

Emily Belmar - *I trade sweat for strength, I trade doubt for belief, and I trade cheerleading for nothing.*

Danny Gregory - *From my own personal experience of being a cheerleader for seven years, I say to become a better cheerleader you need to work hard, which is obvious. I also think you need to be committed and approach every new challenge with a positive attitude and believe in yourself.*

Aly Estvander – *Who inspires me? My mom because she used to be a cheerleader and I want to follow in her footsteps.*

Jade Haynes – *Who inspires me? My teammates and coaches!*

Mariel Singson - *If you're tired just keep pushing.*

Jenna Cartwright - *Always give 110 percent and never stop practicing to become the best cheerleader you can be. Oh, and don't let anyone tell you cheer is not a sport 'cause it is!*

Michele Beauvoir - *Never settle for anything. There is always more than what you know.*

Kenny Vindivich - *Go big or go home!*

Me – Bring all the ideas together and get excited! Take care of your body, take care of your mind and inner thoughts, and this will make you unbeatable! You are special!

Thank you! Please take my advice - you will be glad you did.

Cheer Tumbling Dynamics, Inc.
6846 Thomas Parkway
Rockford, IL 61114

www.cheertd.com
Email: cheertd@gmail.com
Tel: 224-628-5849

A week's nutritional guide

The following is from my personal food diary. With your doctor and/or parents help, you should start making your ideal food list for a week at a time until it becomes a habit.

It took much trial and error before I found the best nutritional routine for me. The everyday results from these choices make it easier as each week goes by. You feel better and stronger, and you look better. You feel good being in control of what you eat, and planning for it. It gives you a sense of control and power!

If you are too young to cook or shop alone, the best place to start is with an older sibling or parent to plan your meals in advance. This way it doesn't seem like so much work. The fact that I cook most of my meals insures that I will like the food and it will be super delicious. I never feel like I'm missing out on anything.

Something that people admire about me is my discipline with my lifestyle choices, and I always tell admirers that there is nothing greater than waking up in the morning and going through an entire day never losing energy, having pep and feeling great mentally and physically.

So I offer you a glimpse at some of my personal menu plans so that maybe you can build yours, with your adjustments, accordingly.

MORNING CHOICES

Oatmeal. Green & ginger root teas.

1 hard-boiled egg, with a big cup of ginger & green tea

1 scrambled egg with green & ginger tea

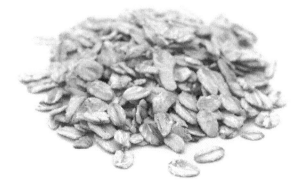

LUNCH

I drink plenty of coconut water, ginger ale (one with real ginger), or filtered water.

Chopped ginger root from my morning tea mixed with 4 cups of frozen spinach, hemp protein powder and hot water with a whole egg blended with some orange or aloe vera juice for maximum energy or papaya/coconut milk smoothie.

Lettuce wrap with turkey bacon, no-dairy mayo, micro greens and turkey meat

Rice with peas and shrimp,

Fish (*white or orange roughy, tilapia, or salmon*) with some sauce.

A whole apple or pear and soup.

Beans, guacamole, salsa verde, rice and chips

I wait 3-4 hours and have 3-4 cups of room temperature water and an apple or kettle popcorn snack.

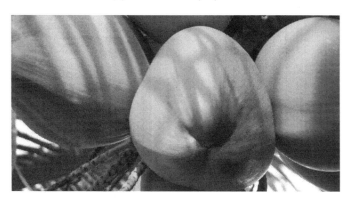

DINNER

Homemade turkey noodle soup

Organic rice pasta

Jasmine rice

A mix and variety of fresh cooked and/or uncooked vegetables

Sea salt in moderation

The leanest cuts of meat

Fish filets

Soy chorizo quesadillas

Whole grain pasta

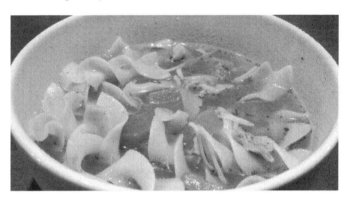

SNACKS

Can be found Trader Joe's or similar specialty grocers

Teriyaki turkey jerky

Kettle Corn Popcorn

Guilt Free Chips

Organic fruits and vegetables (*dried or fresh*)

Chips w/ black bean dip

Vegan Apple strudel

Low sodium chips and salsa

Roasted nuts

Vegetarian chili with kale chips

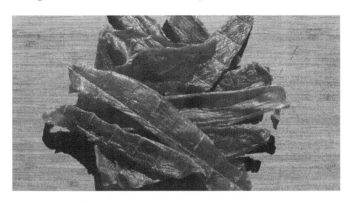

DRINKS

Substitute caffeinated drinks for those with vitamin D (OJ, etc.), green tea and Omega force for long lasting energy.

Fresh fruit and/or vegetable smoothies

Spinach

Papaya smoothie,

Fresh fruit and/or vegetable juices

Beet juice

Orange juice

Electrolyte enhanced drinks

Coconut water,

Aloe vera juice

Smart water

Water, water, water

Filtered water with a little squeeze of fresh lemon

Alkaline water

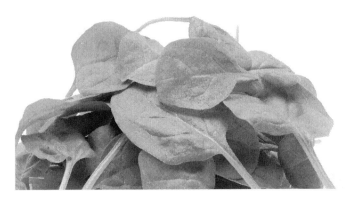

TEAS

I have at least two cups of tea a day.

Chopped organic ginger root with hot water

DoMatcha organic green tea

Yogi teas

Ommune response

Ginger

Super green tea

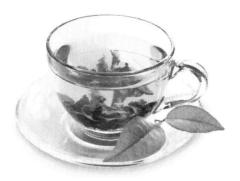

Also be sure that your body is never in short supply of these crucial nutrients…

Calcium, carotenoids, fiber, DHA, garlic, green teas, basil, magnesium, niacin, pomegranate, potassium, selenium, oregano, rosemary, cinnamon, vitamin C, D3 & E, spirulina, Omega force

…to promote great heart health and an overall sense of well being. Eat these foods to achieve that…

red, orange and yellow fruits, green vegetables, white fish, walnuts, pumpkin seeds, real chocolate, avocado, oatmeal, spinach, salmon, mushrooms, brazil nuts, turkey, wheat germ, sunflower seeds, kiwi, hazelnut, oatmeal

Tips for the smart shopper:

Buy a variety of colorful frozen fruits and vegetable for a longer shelf life and this way you always have them available.

Trader Joe's sells wide variety of frozen fruits and vegetables so that you can always have them in hand and not be wasteful.

Prepare meals for the week and freeze so that a quick meal is readily available and food waste is limited.

Side note:

While I do enjoy a tasty snack and a light meal please keep in mind that I do not eat any form of dairy (*save for an occasional egg*). I eat meat three times a week on average and consume more farm raised fish as to not increase Mercury intake.

My nutritional references:

A great website on what athletes should eat:

http://www.ext.colostate.edu/pubs/foodnut/09362.html

An informative nutrition website:

http://www.nutritiononline.net/nutrition-concepts-controversies.html

I often like to read advice from this doctor:

www.DrFuhrman.com

For blood type diets - browse this website and look for your specific blood type:

http://www.drlam.com/conditioncareguide/bloodtypediet.asp?tab=1&condition=bloodtypediet

SUMMARY OF THE RULES

▶ **RULE #1**: It is absolutely necessary to take control of what I put into my body.

▶ **RULE #2:** I must be willing to make a change and new choices. I must be willing to break out of my old habits.

▶ **RULE #3:** Ideally, I will eat five times a day roughly totaling a 2,200 to 2,500 caloric intake. I can make or break my game with the food I eat!

▶ **RULE #4:** Eat well the night before and 3 hours before a practice or a competition to eliminate fatigue, lack of physical strength and undernourished muscles.

▶ **RULE #5:** After the hard work of a competition or workout, I will eat a small meal within thirty minutes of completion to replenish my muscles and energy stores (for better recovery.)

▶ **RULE #6:** Plan Ahead!

▶ **RULE #7:** I can become the best athlete I can with the ultimate competitive edge -- making great daily choices.

▶ **RULE #8:** I will keep my immune system strong.

▶ **RULE #9:** I will have fun! I won't ignore the psychological aspect of fun while choosing discipline in my life.

▶ **RULE #10:** Practice, Practice, Practice!

▶ **RULE 11#:** It is important to challenge myself and be fully immersed in whatever I do to be the best.

▶ **Rule #12:** I will do my research and stay current with rules, trends and competitive moves!

▶ **RULE #13:** Stretch, Stretch, Stretch!

▶ **RULE #14:** I will make myself limitless!

BIBLIOGRAPHY

Block G, Patterson B, Subar A. Fruit, "Vegetables and Cancer Prevention: A Review of the Epidemiological Evidence." Nutr Cancer. 1992 1-29.

Debra Wasserman w/ Nutrition section by Reed Mangels Ph.D., R.D. http://www.vrg.org/catalog/simplyvegan.htm Simply Vegan: Quick Vegetarian Meals (pg 55-58)

Etnier, Jennifer L. Bring your A Game: 2009 (pg 45-67)

Elizabeth Weise "Sixty Percent of Adults Can't Digest Milk" USA Today Aug. 30, 2009 http://www.usatoday.com/tech/science/2009-08-30-lactose-intolerance_N.htm

Erin Beck, "Percentage of Water in Fruits and Vegetables http://www.livestrong.com/article/350652-percentage-of-water-in-fruits-vegetables

Frieden J. ENDO "Diet Soft Drinks Deplete Urinary Calcium" Medpage Today. www.medpagetoday.com/MeetingCoverage/ENDO/20831

Guenther PM, Dodd KW, Reedy J, Krebs-Smith SM. "Most Americans eat much less than recomended amounts of fruits and vegetables" J Am Diet Assoc. 2006 1371-9.

J. Anderson, L. Young and S. Prior "Nutrition For the Athlete 12/10 http://www.ext.colostate.edu / pubs / foodnut / 09362.html

Kemi VE, Kärkkäinen MU, Lamberg-Allardt CJ. High phosphorus intakes acutely and negatively affect Ca and bone metabolism in a dose-dependent manner in healthy young females. Br J Nutr. Sep 2006 45-52.

Kemi VE, Kärkkäinen MU, Karp HJ, et al. "Increased calcium intake does not completely counteract the effects of increased phosphorus intake on bone: an acute dose-response study in healthy females." Br J Nutr. 2008 Apr;99(4):832-9.

Leather S. Fruit and vegetables: consumption patterns and health consequences. Br Food J. 1995 7-10

Lin BH, Morrison RM. "Higher Fruit Consumption Linked with Lower Body Mass Index" Food Rev. 2003 28-32.

Louise Burke "Practical issues in nutrition for athletes" Journal of Sports Sciences http://www.informaworld.com/smpp/title % 7Edb = all%7 Econtent = t713721847 %7 Etab = issueslist % 7 Ebranches =13" \ I "v13" Volume 13, "http://www.informaworld.com / smpp / gotoissue % 7Edb =all %7 Econtent=a790270431" Issue S1, 1995, Pages S83 - S90

Bibliography

Mahmood M, Saleh A, Al-Alawi F, Ahmed F. Health Effects of Soda Drinking in Adolescent Girls in the United Arab Emirates. J Crit Care. Sep 23 2008 434-40.

Massey LK, Whiting SJ. Caffeine, urinary calcium, calcium metabolism and bone. J. Nutr. Sept 12, 1992 1611-14

McGartland C, Robson PJ, Murray L, et al. Carbonated Soft Drink Consumption and Bone Mineral Density in Adolescence: the Northern Ireland Young Hearts Project. J Bone Miner Res. 2003 Sep 18 63-9. Nation Master. Statistics: soft drinks. www.nationmaster.com/graph/foo_sof_dri_con-food-soft-drink-consumption

Ness A, Powles JW. "Fruit and Vegetables and Cardiovascular Disease: a review" Int J Epidemiol. 1996 1-13.

NS Larson, et al "Effect of Diet Cola on urine calcium excretion" ENDO 2010; Abstract P2-198. http://www.endojournals.org/abstracts/P2-1_to_P2-500.pdf

Preedy, Victor R. Nutrition, Dietary Supplements, and Nutriceuticals. chapter 6 pg 63

"Practical Issues in Nutrition forAthletes."Informaworld.com Journal of Sports Sciences. http://www.informaworld.com/smpp/content~db=all~content=a790270431.

Swithers SE, Martin AA, Davidson TL. High-intensity sweeteners and energy balance. Physiol Behav., Apr 26, 2010 55-62.

"Vegetable Nutrition Facts." EveryNutrient.com. http://everynutrient.com/vegetable-nutrition-facts.html

Watson, Ronald R., Gerald, Joe K. Preedy, Victor R. Nutrition, Dietary Supplements, and Nutriceuticals chapter 6 Page 63 (2010)

Weaver, C. M. and K. L. Plawecki. Disease Proof : Health & Nutrition News Commentary-Dr. Joel Fuhrman. http://www.diseaseproof.com/archives/hurtful-food-diet-soda-depletes-the-bodys-calcium-stores.html

FOOTNOTES / ENDNOTES

1 Nutrition, Dietary Supplements and Nutriceuticals. (Pg. 54-78)

2 http://www.svenskmjolk.se/Templates/StartPage. aspx" Lactase tolerant people. (Weise USAToday.com)

3 Reed Mangels, Ph.D., R.D. in the book, Simply Vegan: Quick Vegetarian Meals (Pg. 32-45)

4 Frederick C. Hatfield PhD, author of Fitness: The Complete Guide (Pg. 27-39)

5 http://www.diseaseproof.com/archives/diabetes-diet-drinks-for-preventing-diabetes-no-way.html

6 http://www.examiner.com/x-36995-Philadelphia-Family-Health-Examiner%7Ey2010m6d30-Are-artificial-sweeteners-effective-for-cutting-calories--Are-they-safe

7 http://www.diseaseproof.com/archives/hurtful-food-sodium-and-artificial-sweeteners-linked-to-decline-in-kidney-function.html"

8 http://www.diseaseproof.com/archives/healthy-food-bok-choy-nutrient-dense-and-delicious.html

Made in the USA
Lexington, KY
11 March 2014